Protocols for

Recreation Therapy Programs

Protocols for

Recreation Therapy Programs

edited by
Jill Kelland
along with the
Recreation Therapy Staff
Alberta Hospital Edmonton

Venture Publishing
State College, Pennsylvania

Production Manager: Richard Yocum
Layout Design: Diane K. Bierly
Manuscript Editing: Diane K. Bierly and Michele L. Barbin
Cover Design and Illustration: Sandra Sikorski

Library of Congress Catalogue Card Number 95-60642
ISBN 0-910251-73-8

To the patients of Alberta Hospital Edmonton
who give us daily inspiration.

TABLE OF CONTENTS

ACKNOWLEDGMENTS

Hundreds of hours and the efforts of many people have made this publication possible. The Recreation Therapy department at Alberta Hospital Edmonton is proud to share these efforts with other professionals in the field, and acknowledges the contribution of all recreation therapy staff who assisted with researching and writing these protocols.

The driving forces behind this ambitious and, at times, overwhelming project were Vicki Ryan, director of Recreation Therapy; Janette Engen, assistant director; and Recreation Therapy supervisors Shelley Stasiuk, Deb Bontus, and particularly, Jill Kelland. These individuals deserve distinct recognition. Without their commitment, questioning minds and years of experience, this project would not have been possible.

Thanks and praise is further extended to Roxanne Eyben who designed and produced endless drafts and the final document with such excellence. Michelle Gagnon and Cheryl Robb from the Community Relations department also provided invaluable editorial assistance and support.

Finally, the hospital's Board of Management is thanked for providing the financial support to have this project produced for distribution.

It is sincerely hoped that other professionals and clients will benefit from this team effort.

INTRODUCTION

In the fall of 1991, the Recreation Therapy department at Alberta Hospital Edmonton began preparing for accreditation by the Canadian Council for Health Facility Accreditation in 1993. Upon reviewing the standards, it became apparent the department had well defined and measurable process and structure criteria; however, it was lacking outcome criteria for patient progress. This sparked an extensive review of the procedures and documentation associated with patient assessment and treatment, as well as program planning. Staff decided that in order to produce and document measurable and meaningful patient outcomes, the following components would have to be tailored to suit the hospital's needs: patient assessment, treatment planning, progress reporting, program planning and implementation, and program evaluation.

This comprehensive review resulted in significant changes to the majority of the hospital's therapeutic recreation services. One of those changes was the decision to reanalyze the patient population to determine which areas of functioning most often caused barriers to leisure involvement. These areas became the outcomes to be addressed in treatment services. In a psychiatric population many of these barriers are social because the ability to relate to other people is often impaired; some barriers are physical because leisure skill development has been obstructed; some are emotional because affective expression and experience is limited; and some are cognitive because thought processes are usually disturbed. We revisited our program plan to determine if current programs addressed each of these outcomes. In some cases new programs were added, while others were withdrawn and some changed. Once it was apparent that a comprehensive program structure was in place, the next step was to focus on the specific programs.

After reviewing the current literature and research in the field, staff decided to use program protocols to write up the specific programs. It was felt the protocol format not only gave extensive and vital information about the program, but it also was an excellent means of defining the outcomes associated with a treatment or leisure education program. To ensure each outcome was in fact measurable, outcome attainment scales were written. These scales essentially break the outcomes down into smaller, more defined increments, so that individual patients can be observed and rated. Patient progress is then documented on the scales. Numeric values have been applied to the scales to simplify the interpretation of progress. Reliability and validity measures, however, are not available to date.

For recreation participation programs, protocols were also written, but they do not have separate outcomes. Generally, recreation participation programs are seen to have three common outcomes: to increase the ability to experience fun and enjoyment, to increase participation, and to increase socialization. Therefore, these three outcomes have independent scales which are used (when appropriate) for patients in recreation participation programs.

The implementation of program protocols has had a unifying effect on Alberta Hospital Edmonton's therapeutic recreation service delivery. The interventions (along with supporting documentation) are directed toward assisting patients in attaining outcomes. This will have a positive and long-lasting impact on their leisure functioning. It is these protocols which we are proud to share with you so that other patients/clients can realize these same benefits.

ABOUT THE PROTOCOLS

WHAT ARE PROTOCOLS?

According to Knight and Johnson (1991) protocols are "a group of strategies or actions initiated in response to a problem, issue or symptom of a client."

There are many different types of protocols, one of those being program protocols. Ferguson (1992) presents the following rationale for using a standardized protocol format:

(1) to ensure all elements are included;
(2) to standardize care;
(3) to test specific methods over time; and
(4) to facilitate research.

The purpose of protocol design, according to Connolly and Keough-Hoss (1991), is to write the process and outcome criteria for specific client problems/diagnoses which:

(1) serve as quality assurance tools to measure and evaluate independent therapeutic recreation practice;
(2) serve as references when planning and documenting care; and
(3) serve as instructional tools to reinforce therapeutic recreation practices.

The program protocol format used by Alberta Hospital Edmonton has been adapted from the design suggested by Dan Ferguson at the International Leisure and Mental Health Conference in 1992. While the wording of some headings has been changed, the basic structure remains the same.

PROGRAM PROTOCOL STRUCTURE

GENERAL PROGRAM PURPOSE

This section describes the purpose of the program. It is a statement which summarizes the outcomes of the program, outlining what makes the purpose of this program unique from others.

PROGRAM DESCRIPTION

This section generally describes the program. Whether the program is related to treatment, leisure education, or recreation participation should be noted. The setting and structure may also be described, thereby explaining any element which makes the program remarkable in this section.

DEFICITS THE PROGRAM MIGHT ADDRESS

This section clarifies the types of client problems or deficits that the program might address. The deficits are less specific but broader than the outcomes. This list may also include the positive "side effects" of being involved in the program. (A side effect is defined as an effect that is beyond those outcomes for which it is specifically planned.) Most important, this section should relate to the assessment, highlighting the same areas of difficulty for which the client is being assessed. After viewing this section, the reader would know if the client would benefit from the program.

FACILITATION TECHNIQUES

This section outlines the techniques staff use to attain the program outcomes. These techniques may focus on client grouping, group sizes, communication, specific treatment approaches, props or environments, creating a certain milieu, or any other methods used to reach or fulfill the program purpose.

STAFF RESPONSIBILITIES/REQUIREMENTS

This section is unique to each facility, listing the program responsibilities of each particular classification of staff as dictated by the policies of the organization with regard to job descriptions and other personnel matters. If there is specific staff training required for a program, it should be noted here. After reading this section, it should be apparent what type of staff can conduct, plan and evaluate the program.

EXPECTED PROGRAM OUTCOMES

This section lists the outcomes which a client is expected to achieve in the program. They are stated in broad, general terms. There should be a logical and causal link between the outcomes and the program structure, type, and facilitation techniques. The outcomes should also directly reflect the information included on the client assessment.

OUTCOME ATTAINMENT SCALES

This section specifies how outcomes will be measured. The measures should be written to an appropriate level of specificity, not reduced to trivial detail or written too generally. They should allow for individual differences between clients, but most important, they should be written so as to provide valuable information regarding client progress.

APPENDICES

This is merely a list of program documents. The documents are related to the protocols.

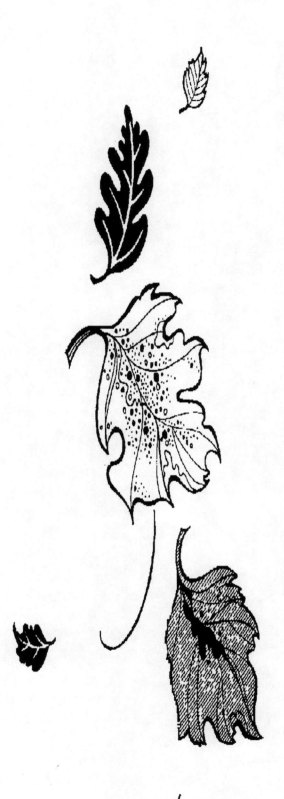

TREATMENT
AND
LEISURE
EDUCATION
PROTOCOLS

PROGRAM PROTOCOL: *AQUACIZE*

GENERAL PROGRAM PURPOSE
To address specific physical, cognitive, and social limitations which interfere with leisure functioning through an enjoyable aquacize class

PROGRAM DESCRIPTION
This treatment program uses structured aquatic exercises, incorporating all aspects of fitness, to assist clients in increasing their physical functioning, social skills, and ability to follow instructions. This is achieved in a congenial atmosphere and to a level which takes into account clients' abilities and which promotes transition into a similar community program.

DEFICITS THE PROGRAM MIGHT ADDRESS
- Poor general fitness level
- Poor general coordination
- Weight control
- Disturbed thought process
- Social inappropriateness
- Low self-esteem
- Lack of ability and/or opportunity to experience fun and enjoyment
- Limited leisure skills

FACILITATION TECHNIQUES
- Group participation
- Experiential learning
- Skill instruction
- Pairing clients whose strengths compliment one another
- Role modeling
- Individual interventions
- Behavior modification techniques
- Providing introduction and access to community aquacize facilities

STAFF RESPONSIBILITIES/REQUIREMENTS
(1) Recreation Therapist
- Program Protocol
- Program Plan
- Risk Management Considerations
- Program Evaluation
- Program Observations
- Program Delivery

(2) Recreation Therapy Assistant
- Program Profile
- Program Observations
- Program Delivery

(3) Recreation Therapy Assistant/Lifeguard
- Lifeguarding
- Program Delivery

EXPECTED PROGRAM OUTCOMES
•Improve or maintain general cardiovascular fitness level
•Improve general coordination
•Weight management
•Improve ability to follow instructions
•Increase social appropriateness
•Increase awareness of community aquacize programs
•Increase ability to experience fun and enjoyment

APPENDICES (Samples)
1. Program Profile
2. Program Plan
3. Risk Management Considerations
4. Program Observations
5. Program Evaluation

PROGRAM OUTCOME ATTAINMENT SCALES

Developed by Recreation Therapy, Alberta Hospital Edmonton

Program: _Aquacize_

Client:_____

Therapist:_____

Diagnosis:_____

Unit:_____

Outcomes:_____

This treatment program uses structured aquatic exercises to assist clients in increasing their physical functioning, social skills, and ability to follow instructions. This is achieved in a congenial atmosphere taking into account clients' abilities and promoting transition into a similar community program.	Assess-ment Date	Review Date	Review Date	Review Date	Review Date	Review Date
A. IMPROVE OR MAINTAIN GENERAL CARDIOVASCULAR FITNESS LEVEL						
0) Unable to participate due to physical condition. 0)						
1) Able to participate in physical exercise 10 minutes. 1)						
2) Able to participate in physical exercise 20 minutes. 2)						
3) Able to participate in physical exercise 30 minutes. 3)						
4) Able to participate in physical exercise for the entire length of the program. 4)						
B. IMPROVE GENERAL COORDINATION						
0) Demonstrates limited use and control of neck, trunk and extremities which results in an inability to carry out the activity. 0)						
1) Demonstrates some limitation in use and control of neck, trunk and extremities. Balance may be affected, and movements may be awkward and stiff, jerky, or slow. 1)						
2) Demonstrates full functional use and control of neck, trunk and extremities; no difficulty with balance or agility. 2)						
C. WEIGHT MANAGEMENT						
0) Regresses from entry level weight. 0)						
1) Maintains entry level weight. 1)						
2) Makes progress towards achievement of personal goal. 2)						
3) Maintains established goal. 3)						
D. IMPROVE ABILITY TO FOLLOW INSTRUCTIONS						
0) Unable to follow instructions. 0)						
1) Requires frequent cues, prompts, or physical manipulation to follow instructions. 1)						
2) Requires occasional cues, prompts, or physical manipulation to follow instructions. 2)						
3) Follows instructions. 3)						
E. INCREASE SOCIAL APPROPRIATENESS						
0) Does not display appropriate social behaviors. 0)						
1) With frequent prompting, displays appropriate social behaviors. 1)						
2) With occasional prompting, displays appropriate social behaviors. 2)						
3) Regularly displays appropriate social behaviors. 3)						

PAGE 1 of 2

PROGRAM OUTCOME ATTAINMENT SCALES

Developed by Recreation Therapy, Alberta Hospital Edmonton

Program: _Aquacize–Cont._   Diagnosis:_____

Client:_____   Unit:_____

Therapist:_____   Outcomes:_____

This treatment program uses structured aquatic exercises to assist clients in increasing their physical functioning, social skills, and ability to follow instructions. This is achieved in a congenial atmosphere taking into account clients' abilities and promoting transition into a similar community program.	Assessment Date	Review Date	Review Date	Review Date	Review Date	Review Date
F. INCREASE AWARENESS OF COMMUNITY AQUACIZE PROGRAMS						
0) Knows where community aquacize programs are located. 0)						
1) Knows cost, time, etc., of community aquacize program. 1)						
2) Participates or has participated in a community aquacize program. 2)						
G. INCREASE ABILITY TO EXPERIENCE FUN AND ENJOYMENT						
0) Does not display nonverbal and/or verbal cues indicating enjoyment. 0)						
1) With prompting, displays nonverbal and/or verbal cues indicating enjoyment. 1)						
2) Occasionally displays nonverbal and/or verbal cues indicating enjoyment. 2)						
3) Regularly displays nonverbal and/or verbal cues indicating enjoyment. 3)						

PROGRAM PROTOCOL: *ARTS AND CRAFTS*

GENERAL PROGRAM PURPOSE
To increase the ability of clients to enhance their independent leisure lifestyle through participation in a learning-centered arts and crafts activity

PROGRAM DESCRIPTION
In a small group or individual setting, clients are taught the skills necessary to complete various arts and crafts projects. Projects are chosen for their potential to develop skills and to challenge clients, while at the same time providing opportunities for success and personal appeal. An activity analysis of each skill is conducted, and the best teaching approach is implemented.

DEFICITS THE PROGRAM MIGHT ADDRESS
•Lack of opportunity to express creative potential
•Lack of leisure skills
•Low self-esteem
•Lack of ability and/or opportunity to experience fun and enjoyment
•Lack of awareness/development of personal leisure resources
•Lack of awareness of community leisure resources

FACILITATION TECHNIQUES
•Activity analysis
•Skill instruction and demonstration, using various teaching methods
•Small group interaction
•Experiential learning
•Individual intervention
•Behavior modification techniques
•Client input into choice of project

STAFF RESPONSIBILITIES/REQUIREMENTS
(1) Recreation Therapist
•Program Protocol
•Program Plan
•Risk Management Considerations
•Program Evaluation
•Program Observations
•Program Delivery

(2) Recreation Therapy Assistant
•Program Profile
•Program Observations
•Program Delivery

EXPECTED PROGRAM OUTCOMES
•Increase exposure to community leisure resources
•Enhance self-esteem
•Increase ability to experience fun and enjoyment
•Increase personal leisure resources

APPENDICES (Samples)

1. Program Profile
2. Program Plan
3. Risk Management Considerations
4. Program Observations
5. Program Evaluation

PROGRAM OUTCOME ATTAINMENT SCALES

Developed by Recreation Therapy, Alberta Hospital Edmonton

Program: _Arts and Crafts_   Diagnosis:_____

Client:_____   Unit:_____

Therapist:_____   Outcomes:_____

Clients are taught the skills necessary to complete various arts and crafts projects. Projects are chosen for their potential to develop skills and to challenge clients, while at the same time providing opportunities for success and personal appeal.	Assessment Date	Review Date	Review Date	Review Date	Review Date	Review Date
A. INCREASE EXPOSURE TO COMMUNITY LEISURE RESOURCES						
0) Cannot recognize/list any community craft resources. 0)						
1) Can list one-to-two community resources (e.g., classes, programs, material/supply stores). 1)						
2) Can list more than three community resources. 2)						
3) Can identify and use community resources on a consistent basis. 3)						
B. ENHANCE SELF-ESTEEM						
Factors: •Neat/clean appearance •Makes three positive statements about self •Smiles •Perceives that people like him/her •Assertive •Positive self-image (makes no self-depreciating remarks)						
0) Problem with three or more factors. 0)						
1) Problem with two factors. 1)						
2) Problem with one factor. 2)						
3) No problem with any of the above factors. 3)						
C. INCREASE ABILITY TO EXPERIENCE FUN AND ENJOYMENT						
0) Does not display nonverbal and/or verbal cues indicating enjoyment. 0)						
1) With prompting, displays nonverbal and or verbal cues indicating enjoyment. 1)						
2) Occasionally displays nonverbal and/or verbal cues indicating enjoyment. 2)						
3) Regularly displays nonverbal and/or verbal cues indicating enjoyment. 3)						

PROGRAM OUTCOME ATTAINMENT SCALES

Developed by Recreation Therapy, Alberta Hospital Edmonton

Program: _Arts/Crafts—Cont._   Diagnosis:_____

Client:_____   Unit:_____

Therapist:_____   Outcomes:_____

Clients are taught the skills necessary to complete various arts and crafts projects. Projects are chosen for their potential to develop skills and to challenge clients, while at the same time providing opportunities for success and personal appeal.	Assess-ment Date	Review Date	Review Date	Review Date	Review Date	Review Date
D. INCREASE PERSONAL LEISURE RESOURCES						
•Increase Leisure Skills Related to Crafts						
0) Cannot complete a craft project. 0)						
1) Can complete a craft project with frequent assistance. 1)						
2) Can complete a craft project with occasional assistance. 2)						
3) Can complete a craft project independently. 3)						
4) Assists others with craft projects. 4)						
•Increase Awareness of Various Crafts						
0) Has no knowledge of crafts. 0)						
1) Has knowledge of one-to-three crafts. 1)						
2) Has knowledge of our or more difference crafts. 2)						

PAGE 2 of 2

PROGRAM PROTOCOL: *BAKING*

GENERAL PROGRAM PURPOSE
To increase the leisure skills and, consequently, the ability of clients to participate in a cognitively oriented social leisure activity in an enjoyable and appropriate manner

PROGRAM DESCRIPTION
In this treatment program, staff create a social, yet structured, environment where clients work cooperatively and assume responsibility for the baking project(s) of their choice. Skills are analyzed and taught through verbal and written instruction and demonstration. The method and level of instruction is determined by the client's ability and level of motivation.

DEFICITS THE PROGRAM MIGHT ADDRESS
•Limited leisure skills
•Decreased social interaction
•Social inappropriateness
•Low self-esteem
•Lack of ability and/or opportunity to experience fun and enjoyment
•Limited decision-making skills
•Decreased ability to adapt to a new environment

FACILITATION TECHNIQUES
•Activity analysis
•Skill instruction and demonstration
•Group participation
•Pairing clients whose strengths compliment one another
•Individual interventions
•Role modeling
•Motivational techniques
•Experiential learning

STAFF RESPONSIBILITIES/REQUIREMENTS
(1) Recreation Therapist
•Program Protocol
•Program Plan
•Risk Management Considerations
•Program Evaluation
•Program Observations
•Program Delivery

(2) Recreation Therapy Assistant
•Program Profile
•Program Observations
•Program Delivery

EXPECTED PROGRAM OUTCOMES
•Improve or maintain baking skills
•Increase ability to experience fun and enjoyment
•Increase socially appropriate behaviors
•Enhance self-esteem

APPENDICES (Samples)

1. Program Profile
2. Program Plan
3. Risk Management Considerations
4. Program Observations
5. Program Evaluation

PROGRAM OUTCOME ATTAINMENT SCALES

Developed by Recreation Therapy, Alberta Hospital Edmonton

Program: _Baking_   Diagnosis:_____

Client:_____   Unit:_____

Therapist:_____   Outcomes:_____

In this treatment program, staff create a social, yet structured, environment where clients work cooperatively and assume responsibility for the baking project(s) of their choice. Skills are analyzed and taught through verbal and written instruction and demonstration.	Assess-ment Date	Review Date	Review Date	Review Date	Review Date	Review Date
A. IMPROVE OR MAINTAIN BAKING SKILLS						
0) Cannot follow recipe and baking instructions. 0)						
1) Requires constant supervision to follow recipe and baking instructions. 1)						
2) Follows recipe and baking instructions with limited supervision. 2)						
3) Follows recipe and baking instructions independently. 3)						
4) Assists others with recipe and baking instructions. 4)						
B. INCREASE ABILITY TO EXPERIENCE FUN AND ENJOYMENT						
0) Does not display nonverbal and/or verbal cues indicating enjoyment. 0)						
1) With prompts, displays nonverbal and/or verbal cues indicating enjoyment. 1)						
2) Occasionally displays nonverbal and/or verbal cues indicating enjoyment. 2)						
3) Regularly displays nonverbal and/or verbal cues indicating enjoyment. 3)						
C. INCREASE SOCIALLY APPROPRIATE BEHAVIORS						
0) Does not display behaviors appropriate for a social leisure activity. 0)						
1) With frequent prompts, displays behaviors appropriate for a social leisure activity. 1)						
2) With occasional prompts, displays behaviors appropriate for a social leisure activity. 2)						
3) Regularly displays behaviors appropriate for a social leisure activity. 3)						
D. ENHANCE SELF-ESTEEM						

Factors:
- Neat/clean appearance
- Makes three positive statements about self
- Smiles
- Perceives that people like him/her
- Assertive
- Positive self-image (makes no self-depreciating remarks)

0) Problem with three or more factors. 0)						
1) Problem with two factors. 1)						
2) Problem with one factor. 2)						
3) No problem with any of the above factors. 3)						

PAGE 1 of 1

PROGRAM PROTOCOL: *BOWLING*

GENERAL PROGRAM PURPOSE
To provide an opportunity for clients to develop the skills necessary to participate in a community-based leisure activity

PROGRAM DESCRIPTION
Clients are encouraged to participate in and enjoy a noncompetitive game of bowling in a community facility, while being taught bowling skills and etiquette, as well as appropriate community behavior and general community awareness.

DEFICITS THE PROGRAM MIGHT ADDRESS
- Limited leisure skills
- Lack of social skills
- Lack of ability and/or opportunity to experience fun and enjoyment
- Social inappropriateness
- Low self-esteem
- Decreased social interaction

FACILITATION TECHNIQUES
- Skill instruction and demonstration
- Pairing clients whose strengths compliment one another
- Role modeling, shaping, chaining, and positive reinforcement
- Experiential learning
- Individual intervention
- Motivational techniques

STAFF RESPONSIBILITIES/REQUIREMENTS
(1) Recreation Therapist
- Program Protocol
- Program Plan
- Risk Management Considerations
- Program Evaluation
- Program Observations
- Program Delivery

(2) Recreation Therapy Assistant
- Program Profile
- Program Observations
- Program Delivery

EXPECTED PROGRAM OUTCOMES
- Improve physical skills required to bowl
- Improve score-keeping skills
- Improve understanding of bowling rules and etiquette
- Improve ability to interact with peers
- Improve appropriate social behaviors
- Increase ability to experience fun and enjoyment
- Enhance self-esteem

APPENDICES (Samples)

1. Program Profile
2. Program Plan
3. Risk Management Considerations
4. Program Observations
5. Program Evaluation

PROGRAM OUTCOME ATTAINMENT SCALES

Developed by Recreation Therapy, Alberta Hospital Edmonton

Program: *Bowling*

Diagnosis:_____

Client:_____

Unit:_____

Therapist:_____

Outcomes:_____

Clients are encouraged to participate in and enjoy a noncompetitive game of bowling in a community facility, while being taught bowling skills and etiquette, as well as appropriate community behavior and general community awareness.	Assessment Date	Review Date	Review Date	Review Date	Review Date	Review Date
A. IMPROVE PHYSICAL SKILLS REQUIRED TO BOWL						
0) Does not have skills to deliver ball. 0)						
1) With frequent prompting, can deliver ball. 1)						
2) With occasional prompting, can deliver ball. 2)						
3) Delivers ball with ease. 3)						
B. IMPROVE ABILITY TO KEEP SCORE						
0) Cannot understand scorekeeping. 0)						
1) Can keep score with frequent staff assistance. 1)						
2) Can keep score with occasional staff assistance. 2)						
3) Can keep score independently. 3)						
C. IMPROVE UNDERSTANDING OF BOWLING RULES/ETIQUETTE						
0) Does not follow the rules/etiquette. 0)						
1) Follows some of the rules/etiquette. 1)						
2) Follows most of the rules/etiquette. 2)						
3) Follows all of the rules/etiquette. 3)						
D. IMPROVE ABILITY TO INTERACT WITH PEERS						
0) Does not interact with peers. 0)						
1) With frequent prompting, interacts with peers. 1)						
2) With occasional prompting, interacts with peers. 2)						
3) Independently interacts with peers. 3)						
E. IMPROVE APPROPRIATE SOCIAL BEHAVIORS						
0) Does not display appropriate social behaviors. 0)						
1) With frequent prompting, displays appropriate social behaviors. 1)						
2) With occasional prompting, displays appropriate social behaviors. 2)						
3) Regularly displays appropriate social behaviors. 3)						
F. INCREASE ABILITY TO EXPERIENCE FUN AND ENJOYMENT						
0) Does not display nonverbal and/or verbal cues indicating enjoyment. 0)						
1) With prompting, displays nonverbal and/or verbal cues indicating enjoyment. 1)						
2) Occasionally displays nonverbal and/or verbal cues indicating enjoyment. 2)						
3) Regularly displays nonverbal and/or verbal cues indicating enjoyment. 3)						

PAGE 1 of 2

PROGRAM OUTCOME ATTAINMENT SCALES

Developed by Recreation Therapy, Alberta Hospital Edmonton

Program: _Bowling—Cont._   Diagnosis:_____

Client:_____   Unit:_____

Therapist:_____   Outcomes:_____

Clients are encouraged to participate in and enjoy a noncompetitive game of bowling in a community facility, while being taught bowling skills and etiquette, as well as appropriate community behavior and general community awareness.	Assess-ment Date	Review Date	Review Date	Review Date	Review Date	Review Date
G. ENHANCE SELF-ESTEEM						
Factors: •Neat/clean appearance •Makes three positive statements about self •Smiles •Perceives that people like him/her •Assertive •Positive self-image (makes no self-depreciating remarks)						
0) Problem with three or more factors. 0)						
1) Problem with two factors. 1)						
2) Problem with one factor. 2)						
3) No problem with any of the above factors. 3)						

PAGE 1 of 2

PROGRAM PROTOCOL: *COMMUNITY LIVING*

GENERAL PROGRAM PURPOSE
To increase clients' awareness of community-related skills and resources through education and active participation in a practically oriented group

PROGRAM DESCRIPTION
This is a jointly conducted Recreation/Occupational Therapy program that addresses eleven subject areas through both lecture and discussion and regular community outings. Subject areas relate to successful readjustment in the community.

DEFICITS THE PROGRAM MIGHT ADDRESS
Clients preparing for discharge may benefit by increasing their knowledge and skills in the following areas:
- Transportation
- Accommodation
- Leisure
- Volunteerism
- Vocation
- Money management
- Social skills
- Social services
- Drugs and alcohol
- Mental health
- Physical health

FACILITATION TECHNIQUES
- Discussion
- Activities
- Pen and paper exercises
- Community outings
- Guest speakers
- Audiovisual materials
- Homework assignments

STAFF RESPONSIBILITIES/REQUIREMENTS
(1) Recreation Therapist
(2) Occupational Therapist
(3) Other disciplines consulted as required for further expertise

EXPECTED PROGRAM OUTCOMES

•Increase knowledge and skills of public and private transportation systems
•Increase knowledge of different types and costs of accommodation
•Increase knowledge of leisure-related attitudes, skills and resources
•Increase knowledge of volunteer opportunities, expectations and responsibilities
•Increase knowledge of vocational interests, aptitudes and community agencies assisting with vocational placements
•Increase knowledge and skills of budgeting, community expenditures and wise consumerism
•Increase knowledge of social interaction skills
•Increase knowledge of social services in the community
•Increase knowledge of alcohol and drugs
•Increase knowledge and awareness of mental illnesses, medication, wellness, and community agencies promoting same
•Increase knowledge of the basic aspects of good physical health

APPENDICES (Samples)

1. Program Profile
2. Program Plan
3. Risk Management Considerations
4. Program Observations
5. Program Evaluation
6. Community Living Program Binder

PROGRAM OUTCOME ATTAINMENT SCALES

Developed by Recreation Therapy, Alberta Hospital Edmonton

Program: *Community Living*   Diagnosis:_____

Client:_____   Unit:_____

Therapist:_____   Outcomes:_____

This is a jointly conducted Recreation/Occupational Therapy program that addresses eleven subject areas through both lecture/discussion and regular community outings. Subject areas relate to successful readjustment in the community.	Assess-ment Date	Review Date	Review Date	Review Date	Review Date	Review Date

A. INCREASE KNOWLEDGE AND SKILLS OF PUBLIC AND PRIVATE TRANSPORTATION SYSTEMS

•Demonstrates Knowledge of Costs Required to Own and Maintain Private Transportation						
0) Cannot state any costs involved with owning and maintaining private transportation. 0)						
1) Can state one-to-two costs of owning private transportation (e.g., gas, insurance, maintenance). 1)						
2) Can state three or more costs involved with owning private transportation. 2)						

•Demonstrates Knowledge of Public Transportation						
Factors:						
•Knows the number for Edmonton Transit or is able to locate it in a phone book						
•Can ask for proper information on phone and remember it or write it down						
•Can find routes on Edmonton Transit map						
•Knows costs of fares						
•Can successfully reach destination by using necessary procedures						
0) Unable to perform any factors. 0)						
1) Able to perform one-to-three factors. 1)						
2) Able to perform four-to-five factors. 2)						

B. INCREASE KNOWLEDGE OF DIFFERENT TYPES/COSTS OF ACCOMMODATION

•Demonstrates Knowledge Required to Find Appropriate Accommodation						
Factors:						
•Obtains information regarding desired amenities						
•Obtains information from landlord about rent, utilities, damage deposit, etc.						
•Knows how to fill out rental application						
0) Unable to perform any of the above factors. 0)						
1) Able to perform one factor. 1)						
2) Able to perform two-to-three factors. 2)						

•Demonstrates Knowledge of Rights and Responsibilities of Tenants						
0) Cannot state rights or responsibilities of a tenant. 0)						
1) Can state one-to-two rights and/or responsibilities of a tenant. 1)						
2) Can state three or more rights and/or responsibilities of a tenant. 2)						

•Demonstrates Knowledge of Items Required and Costs Involved in Setting Up and Maintaining Accommodation						
0) Cannot state any or very few items/costs. 0)						
1) Can state most items/costs. 1)						

•Demonstrates Knowledge of Different Types of Accommodation						
0) Cannot state any types of accommodation. 0)						
1) Can state one-to-two types of accommodation. 1)						
2) Can state three or more types of accommodation. 2)						

PROGRAM OUTCOME ATTAINMENT SCALES

Developed by Recreation Therapy, Alberta Hospital Edmonton

Program: *Comm. Liv.—Cont.*   Diagnosis:_____

Client:_____   Unit:_____

Therapist:_____   Outcomes:_____

This is a jointly conducted Recreation/Occupational Therapy program that addresses eleven subject areas through both lecture/discussion and regular community outings. Subject areas relate to successful readjustment in the community.	Assess-ment Date	Review Date	Review Date	Review Date	Review Date	Review Date
C. INCREASE KNOWLEDGE OF LEISURE-RELATED ATTITUDES, SKILLS AND RESOURCES						
•Demonstrates Knowledge of the Definitions of Leisure and Recreation						
0) Cannot offer a simple definition of leisure/recreation. 0)						
1) Can state a simple definition of leisure/recreation. 1)						
2) Can give an expanded and personalized definition of leisure/recreation. 2)						
•Demonstrates Knowledge of the Benefits of Leisure Participation						
0) Cannot state any benefits of leisure participation. 0)						
1) Can state one-to-two benefits of leisure participation. 1)						
2) Can state three or more benefits of leisure participation. 2)						
3) Can identify activities that could facilitate leisure benefits. 3)						
•Demonstrates Knowledge of Personal Attitudes Towards Leisure						
0) Cannot state likes and dislikes of leisure or reasons for same. 0)						
1) Can state likes and dislikes of leisure, but cannot state reasons for same. 1)						
2) Can state likes and dislikes of leisure and reasons for same. 2)						
•Demonstrates Knowledge of Barriers That May Affect Leisure Participation						
0) Cannot state any barriers which may affect leisure participation. 0)						
1) Can state one-to-two barriers which may affect leisure participation. 1)						
2) Can state three or more barriers which may affect leisure participation. 2)						
•Demonstrates Knowledge of Methods to Overcome Leisure Barriers						
0) Cannot state any methods to overcome leisure barriers. 0)						
1) Can state one-to-two methods to overcome leisure barriers. 1)						
2) Can state three or more methods to overcome leisure barriers. 2)						
•Demonstrates Knowledge of Resources Required for Leisure Participation (e.g., activities, facilities, schedules, cost, equipment, people, transportation)						
0) Cannot identify any resource categories. 0)						
1) Can identify one-to-three resource categories. 1)						
2) Can identify four or more resource categories. 2)						

PROGRAM OUTCOME ATTAINMENT SCALES

Developed by Recreation Therapy, Alberta Hospital Edmonton

Program: _Comm. Liv.—Cont._ Diagnosis:_____

Client:_____ Unit:_____

Therapist:_____ Outcomes:_____

This is a jointly conducted Recreation/Occupational Therapy program that addresses eleven subject areas through both lecture/discussion and regular community outings. Subject areas relate to successful readjustment in the community.	Assess-ment Date	Review Date	Review Date	Review Date	Review Date	Review Date
C. INCREASE KNOWLEDGE OF LEISURE-RELATED ATTITUDES, SKILLS AND RESOURCES—_Cont._						
•Demonstrates Knowledge of Printed Resources Facilitating Leisure Participation						
0) Cannot identify or locate any printed leisure resources. 0)						
1) Can identify one-to-three printed leisure resources, but cannot locate them. 1)						
2) Can identify and locate one-to-three printed leisure resources. 2)						
•Demonstrates Ability to Obtain Leisure Information Using Human Resources						
0) Cannot use a human resource well enough to obtain all information needed regarding a leisure activity. 0)						
1) Can use a human resource well enough to obtain all information needed regarding a leisure activity. 1)						
D. INCREASE KNOWLEDGE OF VOLUNTEER OPPORTUNITIES, EXPECTATIONS AND RESPONSIBILITIES						
•Demonstrates Knowledge of Volunteer Work Opportunities						
0) Cannot state any agencies, etc., where an individual could volunteer. 0)						
1) Can vaguely state where an individual could volunteer or look for volunteer opportunities. 1)						
2) Can state several agencies, etc., where an individual could volunteer or look for volunteer opportunities. 2)						
•Demonstrates Knowledge of the Expectations Generally Placed on a Volunteer						
0) Cannot state any expectations that would be placed on a volunteer. 0)						
1) Can state one-to-two expectations that would be placed on a volunteer. 1)						
2) Can state three or more expectations that would be placed on a volunteer. 2)						
•Demonstrates Knowledge of the Responsibilities of a Volunteer						
0) Cannot state any responsibilities a volunteer might have. 0)						
1) Can state one-to-two responsibilities a volunteer might have. 1)						
2) Can state three or more responsibilities a volunteer might have. 2)						

PROGRAM OUTCOME ATTAINMENT SCALES

Developed by Recreation Therapy, Alberta Hospital Edmonton

Program: _Comm. Liv.—Cont._   Diagnosis:_____

Client:_____   Unit:_____

Therapist:_____   Outcomes:_____

This is a jointly conducted Recreation/Occupational Therapy program that addresses eleven subject areas through both lecture/discussion and regular community outings. Subject areas relate to successful readjustment in the community.	Assessment Date	Review Date	Review Date	Review Date	Review Date	Review Date

E. INCREASE KNOWLEDGE OF VOCATIONAL INTERESTS, APTITUDES AND COMMUNITY AGENCIES ASSISTING WITH VOCATIONAL PLACEMENTS

•Demonstrates Knowledge of Reasons Why People Work						
0) Cannot state any reasons for why people work.	0)					
1) Can state only monetary reasons for why people work.	1)					
2) Can state other reasons (than monetary) for why people work.	2)					
•Demonstrates Insight Into Vocational Interests and Abilities						
0) Cannot verbalize any interests or abilities.	0)					
1) Can verbalize some interests and abilities.	1)					
2) Can verbalize and expand on several interests and abilities.	2)					
•Demonstrates Knowledge of Resources Used to Obtain Employment						
0) Cannot verbalize any resources.	0)					
1) Can verbalize a print resource (e.g., newspaper, manpower bulletin board).	1)					
2) Can verbalize print or human resources.	2)					
•Demonstrates Ability to Fill Out Job Applications						
0) Requires staff assistance to complete a job application.	0)					
1) Can independently complete an application, but not comprehensively.	1)					
2) Can independently and comprehensively complete a job application.	2)					
•Demonstrates Ability to Write a Resume						
0) Cannot write a quality resume.	0)					
1) Can verbalize personal qualifications, but has difficulty putting into written form.	1)					
2) Can independently complete a quality resume.	2)					
•Demonstrates Ability to Complete a Job Interview						
Factors: •Punctuality •Hygiene •Dress •Appropriate nonverbal behavior •Completes answers to questions •Asks appropriate questions •Researches job prior to interview						
0) Unable to perform any factors.	0)					
1) Able to perform one-to-three factors.	1)					
2) Able to perform four or more factors.	2)					

PROGRAM OUTCOME ATTAINMENT SCALES

Developed by Recreation Therapy, Alberta Hospital Edmonton

Program: _Comm. Liv.—Cont._   Diagnosis:_____

Client:_____   Unit:_____

Therapist:_____   Outcomes:_____

This is a jointly conducted Recreation/Occupational Therapy program that addresses eleven subject areas through both lecture/discussion and regular community outings. Subject areas relate to successful readjustment in the community.	Assess-ment Date	Review Date	Review Date	Review Date	Review Date	Review Date
F. INCREASE KNOWLEDGE AND SKILLS OF BUDGETING, COMMUNITY EXPENDITURES AND WISE CONSUMERISM						
•Demonstrates Knowledge of Expenses of Living in the Community						
0) Cannot list any expenses of living in the community. 0)						
1) Can list only rent and/or food. 1)						
2) Can list most necessary expenses. 2)						
•Demonstrates Ability to Balance Budget With Limited Income						
0) Cannot balance budget. 0)						
1) Can balance budget, but some expenses are missing or inaccurate. 1)						
2) Can balance budget adequately. 2)						
•Demonstrates Ability to Use and Balance Check Book						
0) Cannot write checks or balance check book. 0)						
1) Can do one, but not both. 1)						
2) Can write checks and balance check book. 2)						
•Demonstrates Knowledge of Different Types of Bank Accounts						
0) Cannot identify or describe different types of bank accounts. 0)						
1) Knows the names of bank accounts, but not their uses. 1)						
2) Can verbalize names and uses of different types of bank accounts. 2)						
•Demonstrates Knowledge of Proper Use of Credit Cards and Interest Rates Charged for Nonpayment of Full Funds						
0) Has no knowledge of credit cards. 0)						
1) Can state the pros, but not the cons of using credit cards. 1)						
2) Can state the pros and cons of using credit cards. 2)						
•Demonstrates Knowledge of Wise Consumerism						
0) Cannot verbalize ways to be a wise consumer. 0)						
1) Can state one-to-two ways to be a wise consumer. 1)						
2) Can state three or more ways of being a wise consumer. 2)						

PROGRAM OUTCOME ATTAINMENT SCALES

Developed by Recreation Therapy, Alberta Hospital Edmonton

Program: *Comm. Liv.—Cont.* Diagnosis:_____

Client:_____ Unit:_____

Therapist:_____ Outcomes:_____

This is a jointly conducted Recreation/Occupational Therapy program that addresses eleven subject areas through both lecture/discussion and regular community outings. Subject areas relate to successful readjustment in the community.	Assess-ment Date	Review Date	Review Date	Review Date	Review Date	Review Date

G. INCREASE KNOWLEDGE OF SOCIAL INTERACTION SKILLS

•Demonstrates Ability to Appropriately Initiate a Conversation

Factors:							
•Approach a stranger							
•Get another person's attention appropriately							
•Make an opening statement							
•Engage in a conversation							
0) Unable to perform any factors.	0)						
1) Able to perform one-to-two factors.	1)						
2) Able to perform three-to-four factors.	2)						

•Demonstrates Ability to Use Verbal Behaviors Indicating Attention to a Speaker

Factors:							
•Agreeing or disagreeing							
•Paraphrasing							
•Clarifying							
•Perception-checking							
•Use voice effectively (e.g., inflection, clarity, volume)							
0) Unable to perform any factors.	0)						
1) Able to perform one-to-two factors.	1)						
2) Able to perform three-to-five factors.	2)						

•Demonstrates Ability to Use Nonverbal Behaviors Appropriately

Factors:							
•Look directly at speaker							
•Sit/stand upright or lean towards the speaker							
•Comprehend gestures							
•Make supportive facial expressions							
•Maintain appropriate proximity							
0) Unable to perform any factors.	0)						
1) Able to perform one-to-two factors.	1)						
2) Able to perform three-to-four factors.	2)						
3) Able to perform five factors.	3)						

•Demonstrates Knowledge of Different Levels of Personal Disclosure and When to Use Same

0) Does not recognize or use appropriate levels of personal disclosure.	0)						
1) Recognizes different levels of personal disclosure, but does not use them appropriately (e.g., is too superficial or too intimate).	1)						
2) Recognizes and appropriately uses varying levels of personal disclosure.	2)						

PAGE 6 of 9

PROGRAM OUTCOME ATTAINMENT SCALES

Developed by Recreation Therapy, Alberta Hospital Edmonton

Program: _Comm. Liv.—Cont._   Diagnosis:_____

Client:_____   Unit:_____

Therapist:_____   Outcomes:_____

This is a jointly conducted Recreation/Occupational Therapy program that addresses eleven subject areas through both lecture/discussion and regular community outings. Subject areas relate to successful readjustment in the community.	Assess- ment Date	Review Date	Review Date	Review Date	Review Date	Review Date
H. INCREASE KNOWLEDGE OF SOCIAL SERVICES IN THE COMMUNITY						
•Demonstrates Knowledge of Social Services						
0) Cannot state any social services in the community. 0)						
1) Can state financial social services, but not other types. 1)						
2) Can state types of and ways to access several types of social services in the community. 2)						
I. INCREASE KNOWLEDGE OF ALCOHOL AND DRUGS						
•Demonstrates Knowledge of Types of Drugs and Their Effects (alcohol, nicotine, marijuana, etc.)						
0) Cannot name any drug or its effect. 0)						
1) Can name common drugs, but may not know their effects. 1)						
2) Can name several types of drugs and knows their major effects. 2)						
•Demonstrates Knowledge of What Having an Addiction Means						
0) Cannot define addiction; has no insight into own addiction. 0)						
1) Can define addiction, but has no insight into own addiction, or definition of addiction is inaccurate. 1)						
2) Can define addiction and demonstrates insight into own addiction. 2)						
•Demonstrates Knowledge of the Effects of Drugs/Alcohol and How Drugs/Alcohol Interact With Prescribed Medication						
0) Cannot state the effects of drugs/alcohol or how drugs/alcohol interact with prescribed medication. 0)						
1) Can state the effects of drug/alcohol, but not how drugs/alcohol interact with medication. 1)						
2) Can state the effects of drugs/alcohol and how drugs/alcohol interact with prescribed medication. 2)						
•Demonstrates Knowledge of Community Resources That Help People With Addictions						
0) Cannot name any community resources. 0)						
1) Can name community resources. 1)						

PROGRAM OUTCOME ATTAINMENT SCALES

Developed by Recreation Therapy, Alberta Hospital Edmonton

Program: _Comm. Liv.—Cont._   Diagnosis:_____

Client:_____   Unit:_____

Therapist:_____   Outcomes:_____

This is a jointly conducted Recreation/Occupational Therapy program that addresses eleven subject areas through both lecture/discussion and regular community outings. Subject areas relate to successful readjustment in the community.	Assess-ment Date	Review Date	Review Date	Review Date	Review Date	Review Date
J. INCREASE KNOWLEDGE AND AWARENESS OF MENTAL ILLNESSES, MEDICATION, WELLNESS AND COMMUNITY AGENCIES PROMOTING SAME						
•Demonstrates Knowledge of Types and Aspects of Mental Illness						
0) Cannot state any types or aspects of mental illness. 0)						
1) Can name some mental illnesses, but cannot expand on symptoms, causes, etc. 1)						
2) On at least one type of mental illness, can elaborate on the symptoms, causes, treatment, etc. 2)						
•Demonstrates Insight Into Own Mental Illness and Its Treatment/Management						
0) Cannot state own illness, symptoms, etc. — does not recognize/admit having a mental illness. 0)						
1) Can state/admit own illness, but cannot expand on symptoms, treatment, etc. 1)						
2) Can state/admit own illness, symptoms and treatment. 2)						
•Demonstrates Knowledge of Own Medications and Side Effects						
0) Cannot state own medications, their purpose or side effects. 0)						
1) Can state own medications, but not their purpose or side effects. 1)						
2) Can state own medications and side effects, but not the purpose of the medications. 2)						
3) Can state own medications, their purpose and side effects. 3)						
•Demonstrates Knowledge of Aspects Which Contribute to Mental Health						
0) Cannot state any aspects which contribute to mental health. 0)						
1) Can state one or two aspects which contribute to mental health. 1)						

PROGRAM OUTCOME ATTAINMENT SCALES

Developed by Recreation Therapy, Alberta Hospital Edmonton

Program: *Comm. Liv.—Cont.*   Diagnosis:_____

Client:_____   Unit:_____

Therapist:_____   Outcomes:_____

This is a jointly conducted Recreation/Occupational Therapy program that addresses eleven subject areas through both lecture/discussion and regular community outings. Subject areas relate to successful readjustment in the community.	Assess-ment Date	Review Date	Review Date	Review Date	Review Date	Review Date
K. INCREASE KNOWLEDGE OF THE BASIC ASPECTS OF GOOD PHYSICAL HEALTH						
•Demonstrates Knowledge of the Components of Physical Fitness						
0) Cannot state any components of physical fitness. 0)						
1) Can state the components of physical fitness, but does not display full comprehension. 1)						
2) Can state/understand the components of physical fitness. 2)						
•Demonstrates Knowledge of the Requirements and Benefits of Physical Exercise						
0) Cannot state the benefits of exercise, or what an adequate exercise program entails. 0)						
1) Can state the benefits of exercise, but not what an adequate exercise program entails. 1)						
2) Can state the benefits of exercise, and what an adequate exercise program entails. 2)						
•Demonstrates Knowledge of the "Ingredients to a Healthy Body" (e.g., protein, carbohydrates, fiber, fat, water, vitamins and minerals)						
0) Cannot state the ingredients to a healthy body. 0)						
1) Can state one-to-two ingredients to a healthy body and their purposes. 1)						
2) Can state three-to four ingredients to a healthy body and their purposes. 2)						
3) Can state five or more ingredients to a healthy body and their purposes. 3)						

PROGRAM PROTOCOL: *FITNESS*

GENERAL PROGRAM PURPOSE
To increase the ability of clients to manage independently their individual fitness needs, while improving and/or maintaining their current physical fitness level

PROGRAM DESCRIPTION
Clients are consulted regarding their current fitness needs and are assessed on their knowledge of fitness and weight equipment. An individual fitness program is developed using on-site facilities and equipment, while taking into account facilities and equipment available in the community. Once established on a program, clients are introduced to the basics of physical fitness and weight equipment and are encouraged to increase both their knowledge of fitness and their fitness level. Clients are assisted with their program to the level necessary.

DEFICITS THE PROGRAM MIGHT ADDRESS
- Poor fitness level
- Social inappropriateness
- Overweight or underweight
- Low self-esteem
- Poor knowledge of community fitness facilities
- Lack of leisure activity skills

FACILITATION TECHNIQUES
- Individual and small group skill instruction and demonstration
- Behavior modification techniques (e.g., role modeling, shaping, chaining and positive reinforcement)
- Motivational techniques
- Audiovisual aides and handouts
- Exposure to community facilities

STAFF RESPONSIBILITIES/REQUIREMENTS
(1) Recreation Therapist
- Program Protocol
- Program Plan
- Risk Management Considerations
- Program Evaluation
- Program Observations
- Program Delivery

(2) Recreation Therapy Assistant
- Program Profile
- Program Observations
- Program Delivery

EXPECTED PROGRAM OUTCOMES
- Increase knowledge and ability to use equipment
- Increase ability to follow and understand a fitness program
- Maintain or increase present fitness level through an established fitness program
- Increase ability to transfer skills to community facilities

APPENDICES (Samples)

1. Program Profile
2. Program Plan
3. Risk Management Considerations
4. Program Observations
5. Program Evaluation

PROGRAM OUTCOME ATTAINMENT SCALES

Developed by Recreation Therapy, Alberta Hospital Edmonton

Program: _Fitness_   Diagnosis:_____

Client:_____   Unit:_____

Therapist:_____   Outcomes:_____

An individual fitness program is developed using on-site facilities while taking into account facilities and equipment available in the community. Once established on a program, clients are introduced to the basics of physical fitness and weight equipment and are encouraged to increase both their knowledge of fitness and their fitness level.	Assess-ment Date	Review Date	Review Date	Review Date	Review Date	Review Date
A. INCREASE KNOWLEDGE AND ABILITY TO USE EQUIPMENT						
0) Cannot use equipment. 0)						
1) Can use some equipment with supervision/guidance. 1)						
2) Can use all equipment with supervision/guidance. 2)						
3) Can use all equipment safely and independently. 3)						
B. INCREASE ABILITY TO FOLLOW AND UNDERSTAND A FITNESS PROGRAM						
0) Needs constant supervision to follow a program. 0)						
1) Requires prompting to follow a program. 1)						
2) Follows program independently. 2)						
3) Able to identify how the fitness training components (e.g., cardiovascular, endurance, strength, flexibility) relate to his/her fitness program. 3)						
C. MAINTAIN OR INCREASE PRESENT FITNESS LEVEL THROUGH AN ESTABLISHED FITNESS PROGRAM						
0) Regresses from established fitness program. 0)						
1) Maintains established fitness program. 1)						
2) Increases intensity, duration or frequency of fitness program by 10%. 2)						
3) Increases intensity, duration or frequency of fitness program by 20%. 3)						
4) Increases intensity, duration or frequency of fitness program by 30%. 4)						
D. INCREASE ABILITY TO TRANSFER SKILLS TO COMMUNITY FACILITIES						
0) Unable to transfer skills to community facilities. 0)						
1) Able to transfer skills to community facilities with assistance. 1)						
2) Able to transfer skills to community facilities unassisted. 2)						

PAGE 1 of 1

PROGRAM PROTOCOL: *LEISURE EDUCATION*

GENERAL PROGRAM PURPOSE
To develop the leisure-related skills, knowledge, and attitudes of clients to better meet their needs for leisure involvement

PROGRAM DESCRIPTION
A small group or individual program which uses a multifaceted approach to examine the leisure interests, needs, barriers, and resources of clients and which, ultimately, assists clients to plan their leisure lifestyle.

DEFICITS THE PROGRAM MIGHT ADDRESS
•Lack of knowledge and/or awareness of personal resources
•Lack of knowledge of or limited ability to use community resources
•Unsatisfied with use of free time
•Limited actual or perceived activity skills
•Limited leisure partners
•Barriers to leisure involvement

FACILITATION TECHNIQUES
•Individual intervention
•Discussion groups
•Experiential learning
•Lectures and other educational methods
•Pen and paper exercises
•Audio-visual aids
•Discussion/interpretation of assessment tools
•Guest speakers
•Values clarification exercises
•Personal contracting

STAFF RESPONSIBILITIES/REQUIREMENTS
(1) Recreation Therapist
•Program Protocol
•Program Plan
•Risk Management Considerations
•Program Evaluation
•Program Observations
•Program Delivery

(2) Recreation Therapy Assistant
•Assist with program delivery

EXPECTED PROGRAM OUTCOMES
•Increase understanding and acceptance of leisure
•Increase awareness of attitudes toward leisure
•Increase awareness of barriers to leisure involvement
•Increase knowledge of methods to overcome barriers
•Increase awareness and use of personal leisure resources
•Increase awareness and use of community leisure resources
•Increase use of leisure time in a personal and rewarding manner

APPENDICES (Samples)
1. Program Profile
2. Program Plan
3. Risk Management Considerations
4. Program Observations
5. Program Evaluation
6. Leisure Education Pretest/Posttest

PROGRAM OUTCOME ATTAINMENT SCALES

Developed by Recreation Therapy, Alberta Hospital Edmonton

Program: _Leisure Education_   Diagnosis:_____

Client:_____   Unit:_____

Therapist:_____   Outcomes:_____

A small group or individual program which uses a multifaceted approach to examine the leisure interests, needs, barriers and resources of clients and which, ultimately, assists clients to plan their leisure lifestyle.	Assessment Date	Review Date	Review Date	Review Date	Review Date	Review Date
A. INCREASE UNDERSTANDING/ACCEPTANCE OF LEISURE						
0) Does not understand and/or accept the concept of leisure. 0)						
1) Recognizes leisure only as a term; does not have a personal leisure philosophy. 1)						
2) Able to give an appropriate definition of leisure, showing some relationship to personal lifestyle. 2)						
3) Able to define a personal leisure philosophy and incorporate philosophy in lifestyle. 3)						
B. INCREASE AWARENESS OF ATTITUDES TOWARD LEISURE						
0) Unable to identify any attitudes toward leisure (personal or societal). 0)						
1) Able to express some societal leisure attitudes (e.g., leisure should be earned, leisure is a necessary part of life). 1)						
2) Able to express personal attitude toward leisure. 2)						
3) Able to express the relationship between personal leisure attitude and current/past leisure behavior. 3)						
C. INCREASE AWARENESS OF BARRIERS TO LEISURE INVOLVEMENT						
0) Unable to recognize any barriers to leisure involvement. 0)						
1) Able to recognize that barriers to leisure exist. 1)						
2) Able to list personal barriers to leisure involvement. 2)						
3) Able to explain the impact personal barriers have had on his/her leisure involvement. 3)						
D. INCREASE KNOWLEDGE OF METHODS TO OVERCOME LEISURE BARRIERS						
0) Unable to identify methods to overcome leisure barriers. 0)						
1) Able to identify methods to overcome leisure barriers. 1)						
2) Able to implement methods to overcome some leisure barriers. 2)						
3) Able to implement methods to overcome most leisure barriers. 3)						
4) Leisure involvement is not seriously impeded by leisure barriers. 4)						

PAGE 1 of 2

PROGRAM OUTCOME ATTAINMENT SCALES

Developed by Recreation Therapy, Alberta Hospital Edmonton

Program: _Leis. Ed.—Cont._   Diagnosis:_____

Client:_____   Unit:_____

Therapist:_____   Outcomes:_____

A small group or individual program which uses a multifaceted approach to examine the leisure interests, needs, barriers and resources of clients and which, ultimately, assists clients to plan their leisure lifestyle.	Assessment Date	Review Date	Review Date	Review Date	Review Date	Review Date
E. INCREASE AWARENESS/USE OF PERSONAL LEISURE RESOURCES						
0) Unable to recognize/use any personal leisure resources. 0)						
1) Able to recognize some personal leisure resources (e.g., interests, equipment, skills), but does not use personal leisure resources. 1)						
2) Able to recognize most personal leisure resources (e.g., finances, educational level, past leisure experiences), but does not use personal leisure resources. 2)						
3) Uses personal leisure resources on an occasional basis (e.g., weekly/biweekly). 3)						
4) Uses personal leisure resources on a daily basis. 4)						
F. INCREASE AWARENESS/USE OF COMMUNITY LEISURE RESOURCES						
0) Unable to list/use any community leisure resources. 0)						
1) Able to list one-to-two community leisure resources (e.g., swimming pool, park), but does not use a community leisure resource. 1)						
2) Able to list three or more community leisure resources (e.g., swimming pool, park, YMCA, community center, Parks and Recreation department, fitness club), but does not use a community leisure resource. 2)						
3) With prompting, uses a community leisure resource on a regular basis (e.g., weekly). 3)						
4) Uses at least two community leisure resources on a regular basis (e.g., weekly). 4)						
G. INCREASE USE OF LEISURE TIME IN A PERSONAL AND REWARDING MANNER						
0) Expresses total dissatisfaction with current leisure lifestyle. 0)						
1) Expresses some dissatisfaction with current leisure lifestyle. 1)						
2) Expresses that leisure time is spent in a personally rewarding manner. 2)						
3) Maintains a meaningful leisure lifestyle in the community. 3)						

PAGE 2 of 2

PROGRAM PROTOCOL:
PLANNED GROUP ACTIVITY

GENERAL PROGRAM PURPOSE
To provide clients with an opportunity to plan, lead, and evaluate a group recreation activity for their peers

PROGRAM DESCRIPTION
This program provides individual clients an opportunity to develop skills in planning, leading, and evaluating a recreation activity. Clients choose from a variety of recreation activities which are designed to include all participants. At the completion of the program, the recreation therapist meets with the client leader and gives feedback regarding the program. New leaders are chosen each program day.

DEFICITS THE PROGRAM MIGHT ADDRESS
- Inappropriate interactions with peers
- Limited decision-making skills
- Low self-esteem
- Lack of leadership skills
- Lack of organizational skills
- Lack of ability and/or opportunity to experience fun and enjoyment
- Lack of judgment

FACILITATION TECHNIQUES
- Recreation therapist is a resource/facilitator for the client leader
- Client leader takes responsibility for planning and leading the program
- Large group program
- Experiential learning
- Provide constructive feedback and an opportunity for self-evaluation immediately following the program

STAFF RESPONSIBILITIES/REQUIREMENTS
(1) Recreation Therapist
- Program Protocol
- Program Plan
- Risk Management Considerations
- Program Evaluation
- Program Observations
- Program Delivery

EXPECTED PROGRAM OUTCOMES
- Improve appropriate interactions with peers
- Improve decision-making skills
- Improve self-esteem
- Improve leadership skills
- Increase organizational and planning skills
- Increase ability to experience fun and enjoyment
- Improve judgment

APPENDICES (Samples)

1. Program Profile
2. Program Plan
3. Risk Management Considerations
4. Program Observations
5. Program Evaluation

PROGRAM OUTCOME ATTAINMENT SCALES

Developed by Recreation Therapy, Alberta Hospital Edmonton

Program: *Planned Grp. Act.*　　Diagnosis:_____

Client:_____　Unit:_____

Therapist:_____　Outcomes:_____

This program provides individual clients an opportunity to develop skills in planning, leading and evaluating a recreation activity. Clients choose from a variety of recreation activities which are designed to include all participants.	Assess-ment Date	Review Date	Review Date	Review Date	Review Date	Review Date
A. IMPROVE APPROPRIATE INTERACTIONS WITH PEERS						
0) Talks incessantly or does not talk in groups. 0)						
1) Over-talkative or speaks only when directly spoken to during most of the group. 1)						
2) Converses well but is too loud/soft spoken. 2)						
3) Converses well in group. 3)						
B. IMPROVE DECISION-MAKING SKILLS						
0) Totally dependent. 0)						
1) Indecisive. 1)						
2) Indifferent. 2)						
3) Needs some support. 3)						
4) Independent. 4)						
C. IMPROVE SELF-ESTEEM						
Factors: •Neat, clean appearance •Makes three positive statements about self •Smiles •Perceives people like him/her •Assertive •Positive self-image (no self-depreciating remarks)						
0) Problem with four or more factors. 0)						
1) Problem with three factors. 1)						
2) Problem with two factors. 2)						
3) Problem with one factor. 3)						
4) No problems with any of the above factors. 4)						
D. IMPROVE LEADERSHIP SKILLS						
0) Displays no leadership ability. 0)						
1) Displays some leadership ability with constant support. 1)						
2) Displays co-leadership ability. 2)						
3) Leader if encouraged. 3)						
4) Volunteers to lead. 4)						

PAGE 1 of 2

PROGRAM OUTCOME ATTAINMENT SCALES

Developed by Recreation Therapy, Alberta Hospital Edmonton

Program:_Pl. Grp. Act.—Cont_. Diagnosis:_____

Client:_____ Unit:_____

Therapist:_____ Outcomes:_____

This program provides individual clients an opportunity to develop skills in planning, leading and evaluating a recreation activity. Clients choose from a variety of recreation activities which are designed to include all participants.		Assessment Date	Review Date	Review Date	Review Date	Review Date	Review Date
E. INCREASE ORGANIZATIONAL AND PLANNING SKILLS							
0) Unable to successfully organize an activity.	0)						
1) With prompting or assistance, can organize an activity.	1)						
2) Able to organize successfully an activity.	2)						
F. INCREASE ABILITY TO EXPERIENCE FUN AND ENJOYMENT							
0) Does not display physical and/or verbal cues indicating enjoyment.	0)						
1) With prompting, will display physical and/or verbal cues indicating enjoyment.	1)						
2) Occasionally displays physical and/or verbal cues indicating enjoyment.	2)						
3) Displays physical and/or verbal cues indicating enjoyment.	3)						
G. IMPROVE JUDGMENT							
0) Does not display good judgment.	0)						
1) Needs constant advice.	1)						
2) Needs occasional advice.	2)						
3) Displays good judgment.	3)						

PAGE 2 of 2

PROGRAM PROTOCOL: *RECREATION COMMITTEE*

GENERAL PROGRAM PURPOSE
To provide a working committee composed of treatment clients to plan, lead, and offer input on behalf of all clients in recreation programs

PROGRAM DESCRIPTION
This program will introduce clients to a structured meeting format in which they will fill the role of president and secretary. Clients are responsible for making decisions with regard to specific recreation programs and to inform fellow clients of these decisions.

DEFICITS THE PROGRAM MIGHT ADDRESS
- Lack of effective communication skills
- Limited participation and/or involvement
- Limited decision-making skills
- Limited cooperative behavior
- Lack of reality-based judgment
- Limited listening skills

FACILITATION TECHNIQUES
- Facilitate orderly conduct of meetings
- Organize small group
- Encourage participation of all members
- Provide ideas and suggestions on which to base their decisions
- Act as resource regarding hospital policy

STAFF RESPONSIBILITIES/REQUIREMENTS
(1) Recreation Therapist
- Program Protocol
- Program Plan
- Risk Management Considerations
- Program Evaluation
- Program Observations
- Program Delivery

(2) Recreation Therapy Assistant
- Program Profile
- Program Observations
- Program Delivery

EXPECTED PROGRAM OUTCOMES
- Increase effective communication skills
- Increase participation/involvement
- Increase decision-making skills
- Increase ability to participate in group decision making
- Increase judgment
- Increase effective listening skills

APPENDICES (Samples)
1. Program Profile
2. Program Plan
3. Risk Management Considerations
4. Program Observations
5. Program Evaluation

PROGRAM OUTCOME ATTAINMENT SCALES

Developed by Recreation Therapy, Alberta Hospital Edmonton

Program: *Rec. Committee*   Diagnosis:_____

Client:_____   Unit:_____

Therapist:_____   Outcomes:_____

This program will introduce clients to a structured meeting format in which they will fill the role of president and secretary. Clients are responsible for making decisions with regard to specific recreation programs and to inform fellow clients of these decisions.	Assessment Date	Review Date	Review Date	Review Date	Review Date	Review Date
A. INCREASE EFFECTIVE COMMUNICATION SKILLS						
•Verbal Expression Skills						
0) Cannot articulate properly. 0)						
1) Can articulate simple messages. 1)						
2) Can articulate complex messages. 2)						
•Nonverbal Expression Skills						
0) Does not listen or cannot comprehend verbalization. 0)						
1) Responds appropriately to single words. 1)						
2) Responds appropriately to simple phrases. 2)						
3) Responds appropriately to verbal expressions. 3)						
B. INCREASE PARTICIPATION/INVOLVEMENT						
0) Withdraws from group. 0)						
1) With prompting, will participate. 1)						
2) With support, will participate in an assertive manner. 2)						
3) Participates in an assertive manner. 3)						
C. INCREASE DECISION-MAKING SKILLS						
0) Cannot and will not make decisions. 0)						
1) Makes decisions only when given choices. 1)						
2) Makes decisions, but seeks staff approval. 2)						
3) Makes sound decisions. 3)						
D. INCREASE ABILITY TO PARTICIPATE IN GROUP DECISION MAKING						
0) Rejects or resists group decision. 0)						
1) Accepts group decision most of the time. 1)						
2) With prompting/reinforcement, participates in group decision making. 2)						
3) Regularly participates in group decision making. 3)						
E. INCREASE JUDGMENT						
0) Does not display good judgment. 0)						
1) Needs constant advice. 1)						
2) Needs occasional advice. 2)						
3) Displays good judgment. 3)						
F. INCREASE EFFECTIVE LISTENING SKILLS						
0) Unable to attend and/or concentrate. 0)						
1) Attends, but is easily distracted. 1)						
2) Attends and concentrates. 2)						

PAGE 1 of 1

PROGRAM PROTOCOL:
SPORT AND SKILL DEVELOPMENT

GENERAL PROGRAM PURPOSE
To increase the personal resources needed to participate successfully in a variety of physical leisure activities and, thus, increase clients' ability to pursue physical activities independently

PROGRAM DESCRIPTION
In a structured setting, referred clients are introduced to the skills necessary for successful social participation in a variety of sports and physical leisure activities. Clients are also taught the practical skills, rules, strategy, etc. associated with a broad range of physical activities. These elements are taught using in-house and community facilities.

DEFICITS THE PROGRAM MIGHT ADDRESS
- Limited physical activity skills
- Lack of awareness or development of personal leisure resources
- Lack of awareness of community resources
- Limited social skills
- Problems with cooperative behavior
- Problems with competitive behavior

FACILITATION TECHNIQUES
- Activity analysis
- Small group and individual skill instruction and demonstration
- Experiential learning
- Individual interventions
- Role modeling
- Motivational techniques
- Behavior modification techniques
- Use of community facilities

STAFF RESPONSIBILITIES/REQUIREMENTS
(1) Recreation Therapist
- Program Protocol
- Program Plan
- Risk Management Considerations
- Program Evaluation
- Program Observations
- Program Delivery

(2) Recreation Therapy Assistant
- Program Profile
- Program Observations
- Program Delivery

EXPECTED PROGRAM OUTCOMES
•Increase skills in physical leisure activities
•Increase awareness of community resources used for physical leisure activities
•Increase ability to participate appropriately in competitive physical activities
•Increase ability to participate appropriately in cooperative physical activities

APPENDICES (Samples)
1. Program Profile
2. Program Plan
3. Risk Management Considerations
4. Program Observations
5. Program Evaluation

PROGRAM OUTCOME ATTAINMENT SCALES

Developed by Recreation Therapy, Alberta Hospital Edmonton

Program: *Sport & Skill Dev.*   Diagnosis:_____

Client:_____   Unit:_____

Therapist:_____   Outcomes:_____

Referred clients are introduced to the skills necessary for successful social participation in a variety of sports and physical leisure activities. Clients are also taught the practical skills, rules, strategy, etc., associated with a broad range of physical activities.	Assessment Date	Review Date	Review Date	Review Date	Review Date	Review Date
A. INCREASE SKILLS IN PHYSICAL LEISURE ACTIVITIES						
0) Unable to independently participate in any physical leisure activity. 0)						
1) Able to participate in at least one physical activity with guidance and instruction. 1)						
2) Able to participate in at least one physical activity independently. 2)						
3) Able to participate in several physical activities independently. 3)						
4) Able to lead or instruct others in a physical activity. 4)						
B. INCREASE AWARENESS OF COMMUNITY RESOURCES USED FOR PHYSICAL LEISURE ACTIVITIES						
0) Unable to identify where to take part in physical activities in the community. 0)						
1) Able to identify where to take part in physical activities in the community. 1)						
2) With prompting, able to locate and use a community resource for a physical activity. 2)						
3) Able to independently locate and use a community resource for a physical activity. 3)						
C. INCREASE ABILITY TO APPROPRIATELY PARTICIPATE IN COMPETITIVE PHYSICAL ACTIVITIES						
•Overly Passive						
0) Doesn't care to and/or refuses to participate in competitive activities. 0)						
1) Doesn't try to compete. 1)						
2) Tries to compete, but often gives up. 2)						
3) Tries to compete, but occasionally gives up. 3)						
•Overly Aggressive						
0) Tries to win to the point of physically or emotionally hurting others in the group. 0)						
1) Will not finish the game if losing. 1)						
2) Displays physical or verbal outbursts if not winning. 2)						
3) Displays poor sportsmanship if not winning. 3)						
•Appropriate Level of Competitiveness						
4) Understands and engages in competitive behaviors (competitive enough to fit the social group). 4)						

PAGE 1 of 2

PROGRAM OUTCOME ATTAINMENT SCALES

Developed by Recreation Therapy, Alberta Hospital Edmonton

Program: *Sport & Skill—Cont.* Diagnosis:_____

Client:_____ Unit:_____

Therapist:_____ Outcomes:_____

Referred clients are introduced to the skills necessary for successful social participation in a variety of sports and physical leisure activities. Clients are also taught the practical skills, rules, strategy, etc., associated with a broad range of physical activities.	Assessment Date	Review Date	Review Date	Review Date	Review Date	Review Date
D. INCREASE ABILITY TO APPROPRIATELY PARTICIPATE IN COOPERATIVE PHYSICAL ACTIVITIES						
0) Does not engage in cooperative behavior (unwilling or unable to participate). 0)						
1) With prompting, engages in cooperative behavior. 1)						
2) Understands and engages in cooperative behavior (is able to get along with others, is flexible and is willing to accept group decisions). 2)						
E. OTHER INFORMATION						
1) Can participate in a physical activity that requires the participation of one or more people. 1)	**DATE ACHIEVED**					
2) Can participate in a physical activity not considered seasonal. 2)						
3) Can participate in a physical activity that has carry-over potential (to the community or later life). 3)						
4) Can participate in a physical activity vigorous enough to achieve cardiovascular fitness. 4)						

PAGE 2 of 2

PROGRAM PROTOCOL:
VISUAL FUNDAMENTALS

GENERAL PROGRAM PURPOSE
To increase the self-esteem and personal leisure resources of clients, specifically the skills of drawing, watercolor and acrylic painting

PROGRAM DESCRIPTION
This treatment program is designed to accommodate various levels of artistic ability. Clients are taught, through group and individual instruction, the skills to create line drawings and realistic paintings. They are also taught how mood and physical surroundings affect their abilities. Aspects of shading, perspective form, drapery, composition and proportion (using charcoal, pencil, brush, Conte crayons and acrylic paints) are explored. Clients are given time to practice and are assigned homework. Self-esteem is enhanced through positive interaction with peers and staff and through a sense of accomplishment upon mastering a skill.

DEFICITS THE PROGRAM MIGHT ADDRESS
•Limited ability to express creativity
•Low self-esteem
•Lack of awareness and use of personal leisure resources

FACILITATION TECHNIQUES
•Activity analysis
•Various teaching techniques
•Individual intervention and instruction
•Small group instruction and demonstration
•Experiential learning
•Practice skills
•Homework assignments
•Motivational techniques and positive reinforcement

STAFF RESPONSIBILITIES/REQUIREMENTS
(1) Recreation Therapist
•Program Protocol
•Program Plan
•Risk Management Considerations
•Program Evaluation
•Program Observations
•Program Delivery

(2) Recreation Therapy Assistant
•Program Profile
•Program Observations
•Program Delivery

EXPECTED PROGRAM OUTCOMES
•Enhance self-esteem
•Increase skills required for drawing, watercolor, and acrylic painting

APPENDICES (Samples)

1. Program Profile
2. Program Plan
3. Risk Management Considerations
4. Program Observations
5. Program Evaluation

PROGRAM OUTCOME ATTAINMENT SCALES

Developed by Recreation Therapy, Alberta Hospital Edmonton

Program: _Visual Fund._ (painting/drawing)   Diagnosis:_____

Client:_____   Unit:_____

Therapist:_____   Outcomes:_____

Clients are taught, through group and individual instruction, the skills to create line drawings and realistic paintings. Aspects of shading, perspective form, drapery, composition and proportion (using charcoal, pencil, brush, Conte crayons and acrylic paints) are explored.	Assessment Date	Review Date	Review Date	Review Date	Review Date	Review Date

A. ENHANCE SELF-ESTEEM

Factors:
• Neat, clean appearance
• Makes three positive statements about self
• Smiles
• Perceives that people like him/her
• Assertive
• Positive self-image (makes no self-depreciating remarks)

0) Problem with four or more factors. 0)						
1) Problem with three factors. 1)						
2) Problem with two factors. 2)						
3) Problem with one factor. 3)						
4) No problem with any of the above factors. 4)						

B. INCREASE SKILLS REQUIRED FOR DRAWING AND WATERCOLOR ACRYLIC PAINTING

Drawing Skills:
• Form
• Drapery
• Composition
• Shading
• Perspective

0) Cannot demonstrate any of the skills required to draw. 0)						
1) Can demonstrate one of the skills required to draw. 1)						
2) Can demonstrate two of the skills required to draw. 2)						
3) Can demonstrate three of the skills required to draw. 3)						
4) Can demonstrate four of the skills required to draw. 4)						
5) Can demonstrate all of the above skills required to draw. 5)						

Painting Skills:
• Identifying shapes
• Aspects of depth perspective
• Blending
• Application

0) Cannot demonstrate any of the skills required to paint. 0)						
1) Can demonstrate one of the skills required to paint. 1)						
2) Can demonstrate two of the skills required to paint. 2)						
3) Can demonstrate three of the skills required to paint. 3)						
4) Can demonstrate all of the above skills required to paint. 4)						

PAGE 1 of 1

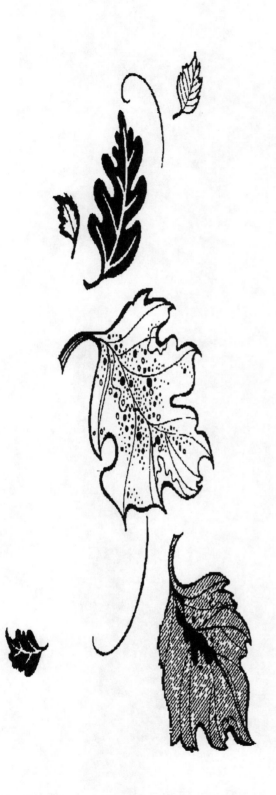

RECREATION
PARTICIPATION
PROTOCOLS

PROGRAM PROTOCOL: *ARTS AND CRAFTS*
(General Participation)

GENERAL PROGRAM PURPOSE
To promote client enjoyment and interaction through creative expression, application of previously learned leisure skills, and self-directed involvement in arts and crafts

PROGRAM DESCRIPTION
Clients who choose to attend this program are provided the materials and instruction necessary to complete various craft projects. Some skill instruction is provided, however, the main focus of the program is on socialization and enjoyment. Clients work individually, while interacting with their peers, and are encouraged by staff to be creative and to apply previously learned leisure skills.

PROGRAM OBJECTIVES
- To provide an opportunity to experience fun and enjoyment
- To provide an opportunity to use previously learned leisure skills in a social and creative arts activity

FACILITATION TECHNIQUES
- Client input and choice
- Individual and/or group projects
- Success-oriented, yet challenging projects
- Limited individual instruction
- Visual aids and samples
- Encourage social interaction
- Encourage creative expression

STAFF RESPONSIBILITIES/REQUIREMENTS
(1) Recreation Therapist
- Program Protocol
- Program Evaluation
- Risk Management Considerations
- Program Observations
- Program Delivery

(2) Recreation Therapy Assistant
- Program Profile
- Program Plan
- Record Attendance
- Program Observations
- Program Delivery

APPENDICES (Samples)

1. Program Profile
2. Program Plan
3. Risk Management Considerations
4. Program Observations
5. Program Evaluation
6. Outcome Measurement Scales
   • Participation and ability to experience fun, enjoyment, and socialization

PROGRAM PROTOCOL: *BINGO*

GENERAL PROGRAM PURPOSE
To provide an opportunity for clients to participate, socialize, and experience fun and enjoyment in a leisure activity

PROGRAM DESCRIPTION
This in-house program is conducted in the same manner as community bingo to allow for the transference of skills. Clients attend this program voluntarily and enjoy the anticipation and excitement associated with this game of chance.

PROGRAM OBJECTIVES
- To provide an opportunity to experience fun and enjoyment
- To provide an opportunity to participate in a passive leisure activity
- To provide an opportunity to socialize with peers

FACILITATION TECHNIQUES
- Creating an atmosphere similar to a community bingo facility
- Individual instruction
- Pairing or grouping clients whose strengths compliment one another
- Inviting guest bingo callers and sponsors from community bingo facilities

STAFF RESPONSIBILITIES/REQUIREMENTS
(1) Recreation Therapist
- Program Protocol
- Program Evaluation
- Risk Management Considerations
- Program Observations
- Program Delivery

(2) Recreation Therapy Assistant
- Program Profile
- Program Plan
- Record Attendance
- Program Observations
- Program Delivery

APPENDICES (Samples)
1. Program Profile
2. Program Plan
3. Risk Management Considerations
4. Program Observations
5. Program Evaluation
6. Outcome Measurement Scales
   - Participation and ability to experience fun, enjoyment, and socialization

PROGRAM PROTOCOL: *BOWLING*
(General Participation)

GENERAL PROGRAM PURPOSE
To provide clients an opportunity for participation, socialization, fun and enjoyment in a community-based recreation activity

PROGRAM DESCRIPTION
In this program clients and staff bowl in a community facility. Staff promote a relaxed, social atmosphere to enhance client enjoyment and participation. Bowling is used as the medium to challenge clients and to practice their skills. Normalization principles are an important component of this program.

PROGRAM OBJECTIVES
- To provide an opportunity for fun and enjoyment
- To provide an opportunity to participate in a community recreation bowling program
- To provide an opportunity to socialize

FACILITATION TECHNIQUES
- Skill instruction
- Foster an environment conducive to socializing and experiencing fun
- Establish a positive rapport between clients and a community facility
- Physical adaptation techniques
- Role modeling

STAFF RESPONSIBILITIES/REQUIREMENTS
(1) Recreation Therapist
- Program Protocol
- Program Evaluation
- Risk Management Considerations
- Program Observations
- Program Delivery

(2) Recreation Therapy Assistant
- Program Profile
- Program Plan
- Record Attendance
- Program Observations
- Program Delivery

APPENDICES (Samples)
1. Program Profile
2. Program Plan
3. Risk Management Considerations
4. Program Observations
5. Program Evaluation
6. Outcome Measurement Scales
   - Participation and ability to experience fun, enjoyment, and socialization

PROGRAM PROTOCOL:
COMMUNITY LEISURE SWIM

GENERAL PROGRAM PURPOSE
To provide an opportunity for clients to experience optimal participation, fun and enjoyment through participation in a community-based swimming program

PROGRAM DESCRIPTION
This general participation program uses a community leisure center to promote enjoyment. Clients who have an interest in swimming attend this program and participate in the activities they wish. The role of staff is to create a relaxed and social atmosphere and to encourage full client participation and enjoyment.

PROGRAM OBJECTIVES
- To provide an opportunity to experience fun and enjoyment in a community leisure activity
- To provide an opportunity for participation in a community leisure activity
- To provide an opportunity to practice appropriate community behaviors

FACILITATION TECHNIQUES
- Individual, small and/or large group unstructured activities
- Client input and choice
- Encourage a social, relaxed atmosphere
- Individual intervention
- Limited skill instruction
- Motivational techniques

STAFF RESPONSIBILITIES/REQUIREMENTS
(1) Recreation Therapist
- Program Protocol
- Program Evaluation
- Risk Management Considerations
- Program Observations
- Program Delivery

(2) Recreation Therapy Assistant
- Program Profile
- Program Plan
- Record Attendance
- Program Observations
- Program Delivery

APPENDICES (Samples)
1. Program Profile
2. Program Plan
3. Risk Management Considerations
4. Program Observations
5. Program Evaluation
6. Outcome Measurement Scales
   - Participation and ability to experience fun, enjoyment, and socialization

PROGRAM PROTOCOL: *COMMUNITY OUTINGS*

GENERAL PROGRAM PURPOSE
To provide an opportunity for clients to participate in and to enjoy community leisure activities while increasing their awareness of the community

PROGRAM DESCRIPTION
Various community leisure experiences are planned and implemented, often in conjunction with clients, in order to incorporate the needs and interests of the client group. Participation is voluntary and staff foster an atmosphere of freedom, socialization, and relaxation. Normalization principles are an important component of this program.

PROGRAM OBJECTIVES
- To provide an opportunity to experience fun and enjoyment
- To provide an opportunity to participate in a community-based program
- To expand awareness of the community

FACILITATION TECHNIQUES
- Participation in community activities
- Client input and choice
- Positive reinforcement and promotion of a positive environment
- Modeling
- Skill instruction

STAFF RESPONSIBILITIES/REQUIREMENTS
(1) Recreation Therapist
- Program Protocol
- Program Evaluation
- Risk Management Considerations
- Program Observations
- Program Delivery

(2) Recreation Therapy Assistant
- Program Profile
- Program Plan
- Record Attendance
- Program Observations
- Program Delivery

APPENDICES (Samples)
1. Program Profile
2. Program Plan
3. Risk Management Considerations
4. Program Observations
5. Program Evaluation
6. Outcome Measurement Scales
   - Participation and ability to experience fun, enjoyment, and socialization

PROGRAM PROTOCOL:
COMMUNITY SOCIAL PROGRAM

GENERAL PROGRAM PURPOSE
To enhance the quality of life of seniors by providing an opportunity for fun, enjoyment, and socialization through participation in a community-based dance program

PROGRAM DESCRIPTION
Seniors attend this community program out of an interest in socializing, music, and dancing. Staff promote enjoyment by interacting with clients. Because this program takes place off site in a more normalized environment the ability to fulfill program objectives is enhanced.

PROGRAM OBJECTIVES
- To provide an opportunity to experience fun and enjoyment through participation in a community-based program
- To provide an opportunity for socialization

FACILITATION TECHNIQUES
- Group interaction
- Individual intervention and attention
- Client input and choice
- Socialization
- Motivational techniques
- Creating a relaxed and positive environment
- Use of a community program and facility

STAFF RESPONSIBILITIES/REQUIREMENTS
(1) Recreation Therapist
- Program Protocol
- Program Evaluation
- Risk Management Considerations
- Program Observations
- Program Delivery

(2) Recreation Therapy Assistant
- Program Profile
- Program Plan
- Record Attendance
- Program Observations
- Program Delivery

APPENDICES (Samples)
1. Program Profile
2. Program Plan
3. Risk Management Considerations
4. Program Observations
5. Program Evaluation
6. Outcome Measurement Scales
   - Participation and ability to experience fun, enjoyment, and socialization

PROGRAM PROTOCOL: *DANCE*

GENERAL PROGRAM PURPOSE
To provide an opportunity for clients to enjoy music and dance while practicing gender-specific behavior and socialize with their peers

PROGRAM DESCRIPTION
This social, voluntary program is designed to create an atmosphere which is as similar as possible to a community dance. Various types of music are played based on client preferences, and clients are encouraged to participate and socialize at a level with which they are comfortable.

PROGRAM OBJECTIVES
- To provide an opportunity for fun and enjoyment
- To provide an opportunity to socialize and practice gender-specific behavior
- To provide an opportunity for creative expression

FACILITATION TECHNIQUES
- Play various types of music
- Play specific requests
- Provide refreshments
- Provide various dance formats (disc jockey, band, karaoke)
- Create theme nights
- Provide ice breaker dances and spot dances
- Role modeling
- Promote social interaction
- Encourage gender-specific behavior

STAFF RESPONSIBILITIES/REQUIREMENTS
(1) Recreation Therapist
- Program Protocol
- Program Evaluation
- Risk Management Considerations
- Program Observations
- Program Delivery

(2) Recreation Therapy Assistant
- Program Profile
- Program Plan
- Record Attendance
- Program Observations
- Program Delivery

APPENDICES (Samples)
1. Program Profile
2. Program Plan
3. Risk Management Considerations
4. Program Observations
5. Program Evaluation
6. Outcome Measurement Scales
   - Participation and ability to experience fun, enjoyment, and socialization

PROGRAM PROTOCOL: *DISCUSSION GROUP*

GENERAL PROGRAM PURPOSE
To enhance and/or restore the dignity and self-worth of seniors by providing an opportunity to share past experiences and achievements and to express an opinion on current world affairs

PROGRAM DESCRIPTION
Clients voluntarily attend this program to seek companionship and social stimulation. A positive and nonthreatening environment is created to encourage clients to share life experiences and other topics of interest. These accounts are listened to with interest and appreciation.

PROGRAM OBJECTIVES
- To provide an opportunity to socialize with peers
- To expand interest and awareness of current world affairs
- To rekindle dormant memories
- To experience companionship, fun, and enjoyment

FACILITATION TECHNIQUES
- Create a positive, nonthreatening environment
- Individual and/or group interaction
- Use various mediums to stimulate memories, feelings and conversation (e.g., newspapers, pictures, objects, music)
- Remotivation techniques
- Positive reinforcement

STAFF RESPONSIBILITIES/REQUIREMENTS
(1) Recreation Therapist
- Program Protocol
- Program Evaluation
- Risk Management Considerations
- Program Observations
- Program Delivery

(2) Recreation Therapy Assistant
- Program Profile
- Program Plan
- Record Attendance
- Program Observations
- Program Delivery

APPENDICES (Samples)
1. Program Profile
2. Program Plan
3. Risk Management Considerations
4. Program Observations
5. Program Evaluation
6. Outcome Measurement Scales
   - Participation and ability to experience fun, enjoyment, and socialization

PROGRAM PROTOCOL: *FRIENDSHIP HOUR*

GENERAL PROGRAM PURPOSE
To provide an opportunity for seniors to socialize and experience enjoyment through various new and familiar leisure activities

PROGRAM DESCRIPTION
This in-house recreation program uses various age appropriate social leisure activities (e.g., cards, games, visiting) to promote client enjoyment and socialization in a relaxed, social atmosphere. Participation is voluntary, yet is encouraged by one-on-one contact and by allowing for client input and choice.

PROGRAM OBJECTIVES
- To provide an opportunity to experience fun and enjoyment
- To provide an opportunity for socialization

FACILITATION TECHNIQUES
- Individual, small and/or large group social activities
- Socialization by staff, volunteers and family members
- Client input and choice
- Individual intervention
- Activity adaptation
- Pairing or grouping clients to promote socialization
- Low staff/client ratio

STAFF RESPONSIBILITIES/REQUIREMENTS
(1) Recreation Therapist
- Program Protocol
- Program Evaluation
- Risk Management Considerations
- Program Observations
- Program Delivery

(2) Recreation Therapy Assistant
- Program Profile
- Program Plan
- Record Attendance
- Program Observations
- Program Delivery

APPENDICES (Samples)
1. Program Profile
2. Program Plan
3. Risk Management Considerations
4. Program Observations
5. Program Evaluation
6. Outcome Measurement Scales
- Participation and ability to experience fun, enjoyment, and socialization

PROGRAM PROTOCOL: *MUSIC*

GENERAL PROGRAM PURPOSE
To provide an opportunity for clients to experience enjoyment in a social-based music program

PROGRAM DESCRIPTION
This social-based music program uses various types and sources of music to create an environment that is conducive to socialization, as well as to individual enjoyment and expression. Clients attend voluntarily and may be drawn to the program by an interest in music or a desire to socialize.

PROGRAM OBJECTIVES
- To provide an opportunity for fun and enjoyment
- To provide an opportunity to participate in a social-based music program

FACILITATION TECHNIQUES
- Small and/or large groups
- Use of live or taped music
- Motivational techniques
- Musical games
- Use of karaoke machine
- Use of client talent
- Role modeling
- Individual intervention and attention

STAFF RESPONSIBILITIES/REQUIREMENTS
(1) Recreation Therapist
- Program Protocol
- Program Evaluation
- Risk Management Considerations
- Program Observations
- Program Delivery

(2) Recreation Therapy Assistant
- Program Profile
- Program Plan
- Record Attendance
- Program Observations
- Program Delivery

APPENDICES (Samples)
1. Program Profile
2. Program Plan
3. Risk Management Considerations
4. Program Observations
5. Program Evaluation
6. Outcome Measurement Scales
- Participation and ability to experience fun, enjoyment, and socialization

PROGRAM PROTOCOL: *PET THERAPY*

GENERAL PROGRAM PURPOSE
To provide an opportunity for clients to experience the benefits of interacting with a pet

PROGRAM DESCRIPTION
Clients voluntarily visit approved pets and are encouraged to walk, groom and play with them independently or in the presence of hospital staff. This program is excellent for clients who have an interest in animals, who respond minimally to other programs, and who have little family support.

PROGRAM OBJECTIVES
- To provide an opportunity to benefit from interaction with pets
- To provide an opportunity to experience fun and enjoyment
- To establish a foundation for developing further trusting relationships
- To provide an opportunity for interactions that are nonthreatening, accepting and tactile in nature (This type of interaction is limited in a hospital setting.)

FACILITATION TECHNIQUES
- Skill instruction in grooming commands
- Positive reinforcement
- Allow client to be alone with the pet(s)
- Encourage client to play with the pet(s)

STAFF RESPONSIBILITIES/REQUIREMENTS
(1) Recreation Therapist
- Program Protocol
- Program Evaluation
- Risk Management Considerations
- Program Observations
- Program Delivery

(2) Recreation Therapy Assistant
- Program Profile
- Program Plan
- Record Attendance
- Program Observations
- Program Delivery

APPENDICES (Samples)
1. Program Profile
2. Program Plan
3. Risk Management Considerations
4. Program Observations
5. Program Evaluation
6. Outcome Measurement Scales
- Participation and ability to experience fun, enjoyment, and socialization

PROGRAM PROTOCOL: *PHYSICAL ACTIVITIES*

GENERAL PROGRAM PURPOSE
To provide an opportunity for physical participation, fun and socialization with peers through a drop-in gym and aquatic program

PROGRAM DESCRIPTION
Using the gym, swimming pool, or outdoor facilities, various physical activities are planned and implemented, in conjunction with clients, to promote optimal participation and enjoyment by all. Attendance and participation is based on client responsibility and intrinsic motivation. Opportunities for safe risk-taking and for challenge are encouraged and provided.

PROGRAM OBJECTIVES
  • To provide an opportunity for fun and enjoyment
  • To provide an opportunity for participation in physical activities which may have elements of risk-taking and challenge
  • To provide an opportunity to socialize

FACILITATION TECHNIQUES
  • Plan and organize various physically-oriented sports and games
  • Client input and choice
  • Limited skill development and instruction
  • Individual and group involvement
  • Encourage a light-hearted approach to the activities
  • Encourage good sporting conduct
  • Explain activity rules
  • Foster an environment conducive to socialization and enjoyment
  • Role modeling

STAFF RESPONSIBILITIES/REQUIREMENTS
(1) Recreation Therapist
  • Program Protocol
  • Program Evaluation
  • Risk Management Considerations
  • Program Observations
  • Program Delivery

(2) Recreation Therapy Assistant
  • Program Profile
  • Program Plan
  • Record Attendance
  • Program Observations
  • Program Delivery

APPENDICES (Samples)
1. Program Profile
2. Program Plan
3. Risk Management Considerations
4. Program Observations
5. Program Evaluation
6. Outcome Measurement Scales
   •Participation and ability to experience fun, enjoyment, and socialization

PROGRAM PROTOCOL: *PUB*

GENERAL PROGRAM PURPOSE
To provide an opportunity for seniors to socialize in and enjoy an atmosphere similar to a community pub

PROGRAM DESCRIPTION
This participation program strives to create an ambiance similar to a community pub. Entertainment and refreshments are available. Staff, volunteers, and family members promote socialization and play a vital role in creating an environment which stimulates optimal participation and enjoyment.

PROGRAM OBJECTIVES
- To provide an opportunity to experience fun and enjoyment in a pub-like atmosphere
- To provide an opportunity for socialization

FACILITATION TECHNIQUES
- Live entertainment
- Socialization by staff, volunteers, and family members
- Theme nights
- Social dancing, sing-a-longs
- Karaoke nights
- Refreshments (including alcoholic and nonalcoholic beverages)

STAFF RESPONSIBILITIES/REQUIREMENTS
(1) Recreation Therapist
- Program Protocol
- Program Evaluation
- Risk Management Considerations
- Program Observations
- Program Delivery

(2) Recreation Therapy Assistant
- Program Profile
- Program Plan
- Record Attendance
- Program Observations
- Program Delivery

APPENDICES (Samples)
1. Program Profile
2. Program Plan
3. Risk Management Considerations
4. Program Observations
5. Program Evaluation
6. Outcome Measurement Scales
   - Participation and ability to experience fun, enjoyment, and socialization

PROGRAM PROTOCOL:
UNIT LEISURE ACTIVITIES

GENERAL PROGRAM PURPOSE

To provide a pleasant environment in which clients in a secure setting may be physically and/or socially active, thereby allowing them to experience an enhanced quality of life

PROGRAM DESCRIPTION

Based on client input, various leisure activities are planned and implemented. Activities may be held on or off the unit, conducted in an indoor or outdoor setting, or be active or passive in nature, depending on the preference and abilities of clients. The goal behind the activities is to promote fun and enjoyment, to provide an outlet for socialization, and to meet the interests and needs of clients.

PROGRAM OBJECTIVES

- To provide an opportunity to experience fun and enjoyment
- To provide an opportunity to participate in various physical and/or social activities

FACILITATION TECHNIQUES

- Individual or small group participation
- Unstructured and/or structured activities
- Client input and choice
- Flexibility in program provision depending on the acuity of clients
- Motivational techniques

STAFF RESPONSIBILITIES/REQUIREMENTS

(1) Recreation Therapist
- Program Protocol
- Program Evaluation
- Risk Management Considerations
- Program Observations
- Program Delivery

(2) Recreation Therapy Assistant
- Program Profile
- Program Plan
- Record Attendance
- Program Observations
- Program Delivery

APPENDICES (Samples)

1. Program Profile
2. Program Plan
3. Risk Management Considerations
4. Program Observations
5. Program Evaluation
6. Outcome Measurement Scales
   - Participation and ability to experience fun, enjoyment, and socialization

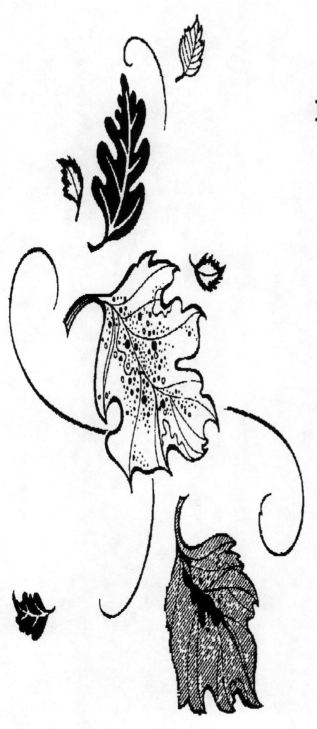

RECREATION
PARTICIPATION
OUTCOME
SCALES

PROGRAM OUTCOME ATTAINMENT SCALES

Developed by Recreation Therapy, Alberta Hospital Edmonton

Program: *Fun and Enjoyment*

Client:_____

Therapist:_____

Diagnosis:_____

Unit:_____

	Assess-ment Date	Review Date	Review Date	Review Date	Review Date	Review Date
INCREASE ABILITY TO EXPERIENCE FUN AND ENJOYMENT						
0) Does not display nonverbal and/or verbal cues indicating enjoyment. 0)						
1) With prompting, displays nonverbal and/or verbal cues indicating enjoyment. 1)						
2) Occasionally displays nonverbal and/or verbal cues indicating enjoyment. 2)						
3) Regularly displays nonverbal and/or verbal cues indicating enjoyment. 3)						

PAGE 1 of 1

PROGRAM OUTCOME ATTAINMENT SCALES

Developed by Recreation Therapy, Alberta Hospital Edmonton

Program: *Participation*

Client:_____

Therapist:_____

Diagnosis:_____

Unit:_____

	Assess-ment Date	Review Date	Review Date	Review Date	Review Date	Review Date
INCREASE PARTICIPATION						
0) Unable to participate because of medical reasons. 0)						
1) Does not participate (is resistive and noncooperative, refuses to stay in area, displays inappropriate behaviors, interferes with activity, is disruptive). 1)						
2) Passive (is a fringe participant, prefers to observe others, requires frequent staff encouragement). 2)						
3) Semi-active (participates with encouragement, wants assistance but does not necessarily require it, needs cues and encouragement). 3)						
4) Active (is responsive, actively participates, makes eye contact, is alert and enthusiastic, appears engrossed in activity). 4)						

PAGE 1 of 1

PROGRAM OUTCOME ATTAINMENT SCALES

Developed by Recreation Therapy, Alberta Hospital Edmonton

Program: *Socialization*

Client:_____

Therapist:_____

Diagnosis:_____

Unit:_____

	Assess-ment Date	Review Date	Review Date	Review Date	Review Date	Review Date
INCREASE SOCIALIZATION						
0) Excessive interaction with others (over initiates, does not respect personal space or nonverbal messages, is loud and/or uses inappropriate or excessive speech). 0)						
0) Avoidance of social contact (does not initiate social contact, ends conversations early, displays uninviting body language, is quiet and/or talks very little). 0)						
1) Does not initiate, but does not avoid social contact (responds minimally to others, maintains a short conversation, has neutral body language, reads and respects others' nonverbal and verbal communication). 1)						
2) Limited social interaction (occasionally initiates conversation; is able to maintain an extended conversation, has warm body language, reads and respects others' nonverbal and verbal communication). 2)						
3) Seeks out and initiates social interaction (often initiates conversation; maintains extended conversation; has open, inviting, expressive body language; reads and responds to others' nonverbal and verbal communication). 3)						

PAGE 1 of 1

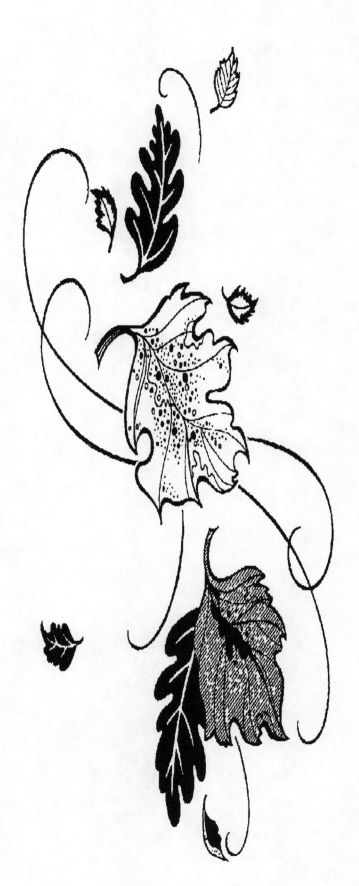

APPENDICES

PROGRAM PROFILE

The purpose of the *Program Profile* form is to outline program implementation details. The programmer must document such details as program time, location, phone calls, and signing-out of keys. This form is invaluable to students, new or temporary staff as it will draw attention to fine details that might otherwise be overlooked.

RECREATION THERAPY—PROGRAM PROFILE

Developed by Recreation Therapy, Alberta Hospital Edmonton

Program:_____ Staff:_____

Unit:_____ _____

DAYS	TIME(S)	LOCATION(S)
_____	FROM_____ TO_____	_____
_____	FROM_____ TO_____	_____
_____	FROM_____ TO_____	_____

Transportation:_____

Keys To Be Signed Out:_____

_____

Phone Units:

   □ Yes   □ No

Reason for Call:_____

Funding Arrangements:_____

_____

Escort Patient(s) to Program:

   □ Yes   □ No

Location to Meet Patient(s):_____

_____

ACTIVITY PLAN (brief overview of activity):_____

_____
_____
_____
_____
_____
_____
_____
_____
_____
_____
_____
_____

ACTIVITIES:_____

_____
_____
_____
_____
_____

Escort Patient(s) from Program:

   □ Yes   □ No

Method of Recording Attendance:_____

_____

Patient/Program Cautions:_____

_____
_____
_____

PROGRAM PLAN

The *Program Plan* form is a vital part of program planning because it allows the therapist to describe how each outcome will be addressed. The format used is taken from Peterson and Gunn (1984). For each program outcome, the content and process are identified. The content is written after a task analysis of the specified outcome.

As stated by Peterson and Gunn (1984), "several factors must be considered in the development and specification of content. The designer must continuously be aware of the type of clients for whom the program is intended." Furthermore, "age characteristics, the size of the intended group, the availability of resources (e.g., supplies, equipment, facilities), and the length of the program will all play an important role in determining the level and amount of content that is appropriate."

In summary, content can be viewed as *what* is going to occur in the program or *what* needs to be done to achieve the outcome.

The process of the program plan is the *how* of the program. Peterson and Gunn say the "process refers to the way the content is presented to the clients." It is in the process that the programmer gives more detail as to the facilitation techniques which will be used to achieve the outcomes. The process specifies what the programmer will do, but it may also make reference to client expectations. For example, if clients are involved in decision-making or in planning a particular activity, these facts would be stated here.

(For more information on writing content and process, please refer to Peterson and Gunn, pp. 113 to 118.)

RECREATION THERAPY—SAMPLE PROGRAM PLAN

Developed by Recreation Therapy, Alberta Hospital Edmonton

Program: _Gym Activities_

Outcome: _Increase Cooperative Behaviors*_

CONTENT	PROCESS

A common disturbance associated with major psychiatric illnesses is the inability to work with others. In schizophrenia this may be due to a disturbance in one's sense of self. In a mood disorder there may be either a marked increase or decrease in sociability. Disturbances in behavior, as a result of organic illnesses or a personality disorder, may also impair an individual's ability to cooperate.
 	
Cooperation entails the concepts of sharing, contributing toward the attainment of a group goal, providing emotional support to others, and engaging in assertive rather than passive or aggressive behaviors.
 	
There are many gym activities and sports which involve or develop cooperative skills. A program which incorporates these activities and which is facilitated adequately can assist individuals in improving their cooperative behavior.
	Plan activities which have a cooperative element (e.g., team sports, cooperative games, initiative tasks).
	
	Observe the ability of individuals to cooperate.
	
	Encourage cooperative behavior through:
	    •group interventions—good teamwork, pass the ball, etc.
	    •role modeling of good cooperative behavior
	    •individual interventions (if an individual is having difficulty cooperating):
	        -point out difficulties
	        -praise positive cooperative behavior
	        -suggest changes in behavior
	
	Individuals with particular difficulties may also be given a role such as referee or captain which places an even greater emphasis on the need to cooperate.

(*Note: The same documentation is required for each program outcome.)

RISK MANAGEMENT CONSIDERATIONS

It is important for the programmer to identify the potential risks associated with a program, as well as to project all possible means of reducing the frequency and/or severity of the risks. The *Risk Management Considerations* form allows the programmer to document these potential risks. The programmer notes whether the program is high, medium or low risk. Risks to be considered include obvious ones such as client injury and subtle ones such as loss of, or damage to, equipment.

The form features one portion of the department's risk management plan and must be completed for each program.

RECREATION THERAPY—PROGRAM PLANNING
RISK MANAGEMENT CONSIDERATIONS

Developed by Recreation Therapy, Alberta Hospital Edmonton

Program:_____ Unit:_____
_____ Date:_____

RISK LEVEL: Activities conducted in this program are considered:
- ☐ HIGH RISK   Precautions must be addressed to prevent injury/loss.
- ☐ MEDIUM RISK   Precautions must be addressed to prevent injury/loss.
- ☐ LOW RISK   Precautions may be addressed to prevent injury/loss.

PROPENSITIES AND RISKS

1. List any propensities which would exclude a patient from participating in this program (e.g., aggression, heart condition, privilege level, elopement risk).

   a._____
   b._____
   c._____
   d._____
   e._____

2. Equipment, supplies, and/or environmental risks include (check all those which apply):

   - ☐ toxic materials
   - ☐ sharps
   - ☐ infection control
   - ☐ water
   - ☐ explosive/flammable materials
   - ☐ equipment/activity which requires specific instruction for safety
   - ☐ activity requires appropriate safety equipment
   - ☐ objects which may be used as weapons
   - ☐ none of the above

OTHER RISKS (please specify):

_____
_____

RATIO
Suggested staff/patient ratio to ensure safety is:

☐ patients for   ☐ staff.

STAFF SKILLS: Staff conducting this program should possess the following skills to reduce the possibility or severity of an injury (e.g., knowledge of safe use of universal gym):

1._____
2._____
3._____

MANAGEMENT OF RISKS: The primary risks associated with this program are addressed by:

RISK	MANAGED THROUGH
1._____	_____
2._____	_____
3._____	_____

PROGRAM OBSERVATIONS

The purpose of the *Program Observations* form is to record the programmer's remarks about the program. Worthy of note are issues (such as the success of a particular facilitation technique), changes that need to be made, comments on resources, or anything else that has impacted the program. These observations help the programmer to reflect on past programs and assist students, new staff or temporary staff to familiarize themselves with the program.

RECREATION THERAPY
PROGRAM OBSERVATIONS

Developed by Recreation Therapy, Alberta Hospital Edmonton

Program:_____

Unit:_____

Recreation Therapy Staff:_____

Frequency of Entries:_____

DATE	PROGRAM OBSERVATION

PATIENT PROGRAM EVALUATION

Patients are asked to complete the *Patient Program Evaluation* form at intervals which are predetermined by the department. Patients evaluate several programs at a time by writing the name of each program they attend in the boxes across the top of the form and by answering the questions for each program.

The form is divided into three sections: *Program Resources*, referring to the mechanics of the program; *Program Content*, referring to what occurs in the program; and *Program Benefits*, referring to the benefits the patient derives from the program. (This section has not been rewritten since the development of the protocols and outcome measures. Once rewritten, this section will more accurately reflect the specific program outcomes.)

This evaluation format allows for easy comparison of programs and assists the programmer to identify which program aspects patients consider to be good and which could benefit from changes.

The two forms following the evaluation tool are forms which the programmer may use to summarize program evaluations. Recorded on the form are the mean scores for each of the three areas evaluated, as well as problems with equipment, reasons why patients attend programs, and general comments. The second summary form has space for the programmer to comment on each area evaluated.

REC. THERAPY—PATIENT PROGRAM EVALUATION

Developed by Recreation Therapy, Alberta Hospital Edmonton

Unit:_____

Date:_____

Length of Time in Rec.

Programs:_____

5 - SA (Strongly Agree) 4 - A (Agree) 3 - N (Neither Agree Nor Disagree) 2 - D (Disagree) 1 - SD (Strongly Disagree)	PROGRAMS					
	SA A N D SD	SA A N D SD	SA A N D SD	SA A N D SD	SA A N D SD	SA A N D SD

PROGRAM RESOURCES:

Please circle the number which describes your level of agreement with each statement.

1. The number of Recreation Therapy programs available to me is adequate.	5 4 3 2 1	5 4 3 2 1	5 4 3 2 1	5 4 3 2 1	5 4 3 2 1	5 4 3 2 1
2. The number of staff in Recreation Therapy programs is sufficient.	5 4 3 2 1	5 4 3 2 1	5 4 3 2 1	5 4 3 2 1	5 4 3 2 1	5 4 3 2 1
3. The indoor facilities used for Recreation Therapy programs are acceptable.	5 4 3 2 1	5 4 3 2 1	5 4 3 2 1	5 4 3 2 1	5 4 3 2 1	5 4 3 2 1
4. The equipment used for Recreation Therapy programs is adequate.	5 4 3 2 1	5 4 3 2 1	5 4 3 2 1	5 4 3 2 1	5 4 3 2 1	5 4 3 2 1
5. The cost of Recreation Therapy programs, if applicable, is reasonable.	5 4 3 2 1	5 4 3 2 1	5 4 3 2 1	5 4 3 2 1	5 4 3 2 1	5 4 3 2 1

6. Please circle the problem areas (you may circle as many as are applicable):
   a. the condition of equipment (i.e., broken, worn-out)
   b. the quantity of equipment
   c. the size of equipment
   d. the quality of equipment
   e. the availability of equipment

OTHER COMMENTS:

_____
_____
_____
_____
_____
_____
_____
_____
_____
_____
_____
_____

REC. THERAPY—PATIENT PROGRAM EVALUATION

Developed by Recreation Therapy, Alberta Hospital Edmonton

Unit:_____

Date:_____

Length of Time in Rec.

Programs:_____

5 - SA (Strongly Agree) 4 - A (Agree) 3 - N (Neither Agree Nor Disagree) 2 - D (Disagree) 1 - SD (Strongly Disagree)	PROGRAMS					
	SA A N D SD	SA A N D SD	SA A N D SD	SA A N D SD	SA A N D SD	SA A N D SD

PROGRAM CONTENT:

Please circle the number which describes your level of agreement with each statement.

1. The Recreation Therapist/Assistant appears genuinely interested in the quality of the programs.	5 4 3 2 1	5 4 3 2 1	5 4 3 2 1	5 4 3 2 1	5 4 3 2 1	5 4 3 2 1
2. I have the opportunity to offer suggestions regarding programs.	5 4 3 2 1	5 4 3 2 1	5 4 3 2 1	5 4 3 2 1	5 4 3 2 1	5 4 3 2 1
3. The Recreation Therapist/Assistant allows me to develop my leadership skills during programs.	5 4 3 2 1	5 4 3 2 1	5 4 3 2 1	5 4 3 2 1	5 4 3 2 1	5 4 3 2 1
4. There is a good variety of activities available in recreation programs.	5 4 3 2 1	5 4 3 2 1	5 4 3 2 1	5 4 3 2 1	5 4 3 2 1	5 4 3 2 1
5. The size of groups in programs is appropriate.	5 4 3 2 1	5 4 3 2 1	5 4 3 2 1	5 4 3 2 1	5 4 3 2 1	5 4 3 2 1
6. I enjoy it when staff participate in programs with me.	5 4 3 2 1	5 4 3 2 1	5 4 3 2 1	5 4 3 2 1	5 4 3 2 1	5 4 3 2 1
7. I enjoy programs that are cooperative in nature.	5 4 3 2 1	5 4 3 2 1	5 4 3 2 1	5 4 3 2 1	5 4 3 2 1	5 4 3 2 1
8. I enjoy programs that have a competitive element.	5 4 3 2 1	5 4 3 2 1	5 4 3 2 1	5 4 3 2 1	5 4 3 2 1	5 4 3 2 1

What other activities or programs would you like to have made available to you?

_____

_____

_____

OTHER COMMENTS:

_____

_____

_____

_____

_____

REC. THERAPY—PATIENT PROGRAM EVALUATION
Developed by Recreation Therapy, Alberta Hospital Edmonton

Unit:_____

Date:_____

Length of Time in Rec.

Programs:_____

5 - SA (Strongly Agree) 4 - A (Agree) 3 - N (Neither Agree Nor Disagree) 2 - D (Disagree) 1 - SD (Strongly Disagree)	PROGRAMS					
	SA A N D SD	SA A N D SD	SA A N D SD	SA A N D SD	SA A N D SD	SA A N D SD

PROGRAM BENEFITS:
Please circle the number which describes your level of agreement with each statement.

1. I benefit from being involved in Recreation Therapy programs.	5 4 3 2 1	5 4 3 2 1	5 4 3 2 1	5 4 3 2 1	5 4 3 2 1	5 4 3 2 1
2. The programs help me physically.	5 4 3 2 1	5 4 3 2 1	5 4 3 2 1	5 4 3 2 1	5 4 3 2 1	5 4 3 2 1
3. The programs allow me to practice my social skills.	5 4 3 2 1	5 4 3 2 1	5 4 3 2 1	5 4 3 2 1	5 4 3 2 1	5 4 3 2 1
4. The programs allow me to express my emotions.	5 4 3 2 1	5 4 3 2 1	5 4 3 2 1	5 4 3 2 1	5 4 3 2 1	5 4 3 2 1
5. The programs help me to feel better about myself.	5 4 3 2 1	5 4 3 2 1	5 4 3 2 1	5 4 3 2 1	5 4 3 2 1	5 4 3 2 1
6. I can apply what I learn in recreation programs to other areas of my life.	5 4 3 2 1	5 4 3 2 1	5 4 3 2 1	5 4 3 2 1	5 4 3 2 1	5 4 3 2 1

7. I attend recreation programs because (please circle a, b or c):
   a. I want to attend.
   b. I have to attend.
   c. I have to attend, but I enjoy the program.

OTHER COMMENTS:

_____

_____

_____

_____

_____

_____

_____

_____

_____

_____

_____

_____

_____

PAGE 3 of 3

RECREATION THERAPY PATIENT PROGRAM EVALUATION SUMMARY

Developed by Recreation Therapy, Alberta Hospital Edmonton

Evaluation Date:_____

	PROGRAMS					
PROGRAM RESOURCES	/25	/25	/25	/25	/25	/25
PROGRAM CONTENT	/40	/40	/40	/40	/40	/40
PROGRAM BENEFITS	/30	/30	/30	/30	/30	/30

REASONS FOR ATTENDING:

_____ Want to attend

_____ Have to attend

_____ Have to attend, but enjoy the program

EQUIPMENT PROBLEM AREAS:

_____ Condition   _____ Availability

_____ Quality   _____ Size

_____ Quantity

OTHER COMMENTS:

_____
_____
_____
_____
_____
_____
_____
_____
_____
_____
_____
_____
_____
_____
_____
_____
_____

RECREATION THERAPY
PROGRAM EVALUATION SUMMARY

Developed by Recreation Therapy, Alberta Hospital Edmonton

Program(s) Evaluted:_____

Date:_____

Provide a written summary in each of the areas evaluated. Summarize patient evaluations, staff evaluations and your comments about the program.

PROGRAM RESOURCES:_____
_____
_____
_____
_____
_____

PROGRAM CONTENT:_____
_____
_____
_____
_____
_____

PROGRAM BENEFITS:_____
_____
_____
_____
_____
_____

SUMMARY AND RECOMMENDATIONS:_____
_____
_____
_____
_____
_____

RECREATION THERAPY—PROGRAM REFERRAL

Developed by Recreation Therapy, Alberta Hospital Edmonton

Program Name:_____

Patient Name:_____

Therapist:_____

Out-Patient Home Phone:_____

Unit Phone:_____

Doctor:_____

DIAGNOSIS:_____

_____

_____

CONCERNS:_____

_____

_____

_____

_____

_____

_____

_____

APPROACHES:_____

_____

_____

_____

_____

_____

_____

_____

Date Completed:_____

Signature:_____

Recreation Therapist/Assistant

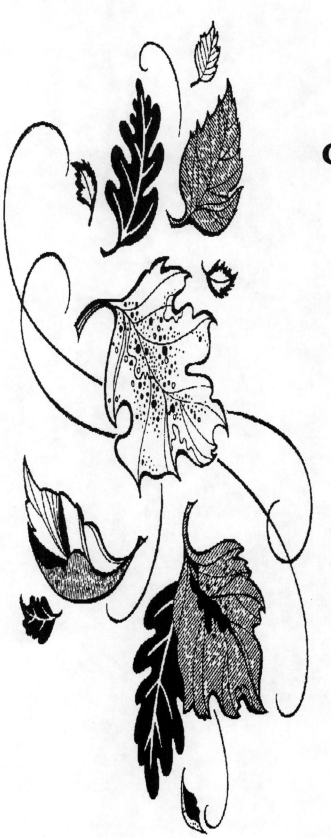

RESOURCES
AND
CONTRIBUTORS

RESOURCES

burlingame, j. and Blashko, T. M. (Eds.). (1990). *Assessment tools for recreation therapy*. Seattle, WA: Frontier.

Connolly, P. and Keogh-Hoss, M. A. (1991). The development and use of intervention protocols in therapeutic recreation: Documentation field-based practices. In B. Riley (Ed.), *Quality Management: Applications for Therapeutic Recreation* (pp. 117-136). State College, PA: Venture Publishing, Inc.

Dattilo, J. and Murphy, W. D. (1991). *Leisure education program planning: A systematic approach*. State College, PA: Venture Publishing, Inc.

Ferguson, D. (1992, July). Recreation therapy protocols. International Conference on Leisure and Mental Health, Salt Lake City, UT.

Knight, L. and Johnson, D. (1991). Therapeutic recreation protocols: Client problem centered approach. In B. Riley (Ed.), *Quality Management Applications for Therapeutic Recreation* (pp. 137-147). State College, PA: Venture Publishing, Inc.

Olsson, R. (1990). Ohio leisure skills scales on normal functioning. In j. burlingame and T. M. Balshko (Eds.), *Assessment tools for recreational therapy* (pp. 175-184). Seattle, WA: Frontier.

Parker, R. A., Ellison, C. H., Kirby, T. F., and Short, M. J. (1990). Comprehensive evaluation in recreational therapy — Psych/Behavioral. In j. burlingame and T. M. Blashko (Eds.), *Assessment tools for recreational therapy* (pp. 107-116). Seattle, WA: Frontier.

Peterson, C. A., Dunn, J., and Carruthers, C. (1990). Functional assessment of characteristics for therapeutic recreation. In j. burlingame and T. M. Blashko (Eds.), *Assessment tools for recreational therapy* (pp. 117-127). Seattle, WA: Frontier.

Peterson, C. A. and Gunn, S. L. (1984). *Therapeutic recreation program design principles and procedures* (2nd ed.). Englewood Cliffs, NJ: Prentice-Hall.

Riley, B. (Ed.). (1991). *Quality management applications for therapeutic recreation*. State College, PA: Venture Publishing, Inc.

CONTRIBUTORS

The editor of this publication, **Jill Kelland**, graduated in 1986 from the University of Alberta with a Bachelor of Arts in Recreation Administration with a major in Special Populations. She then received her Masters of Science Degree in Therapeutic Recreation from the University of Wisconsin—LaCrosse in 1992. Jill worked for two years in acute psychiatry and since 1988 has worked in forensic psychiatry as a recreation therapist and recreation therapy supervisor.

Debbie Bontus graduated in 1982 from the University of Alberta with a Bachelor of Education with a specialization in adapted physical education and administration. She worked for ten years at Alberta Hospital Edmonton as a recreation therapist and later as a supervisor in the acute psychiatry service. Currently, Deb is employed as a recreation therapist at the Glenrose Rehabilitation Hospital with the amputee and rheumatology programs.

Janette Engen graduated in 1982 from the University of Manitoba with a Bachelor of Physical Education for Special Populations and an Education Certificate. Over her twelve years at Alberta Hospital Edmonton, Janette initially worked as a recreation therapy assistant, then a supervisor and the assistant director of the recreation therapy department. Currently, she is the recreation facilities coordinator.

Rosalie Karwandy graduated in 1990 with distinction from the University of Alberta with a Bachelor of Science in Occupational Therapy. Since graduation Rosalie has worked in the forensic psychiatry unit at Alberta Hospital and has pioneered several joint programs in projects with recreation therapy staff with which she has worked. Her contribution to this publication was on the Community Living Protocol, a joint Recreation Therapy and Occupational Therapy program which was highly successful for forensic rehabilitation patients and has served as a model for several other joint programs throughout the hospital.

Deanna LeSage graduated in 1990 from the University of Alberta with a Bachelor of Arts in Recreation Administration with a major in Special Populations. Deanna has worked as a recreation therapist at Alberta Hospital Edmonton for the past four years, two years in the acute psychiatry service and two years on the young offenders unit.

Cathy McAlear graduated with a diploma in Community Leadership Training from Dawson College in Montreal, Quebec. She then received her Bachelor of Arts in Recreation Administration from the University of Alberta in 1986. Cathy has worked with seniors, youth, and the forensic population over the course of her career in recreation therapy. Her most recent challenge is as a community recreation therapist where she is developing a day program for adults with mental health concerns.

Terry Neumann graduated from the University of Alberta with a Bachelor of Arts in Recreation Administration with a major in Special Populations. She also has one year's training in the Psychosocial Rehabilitation Model from Boston, Massachusettes. Terry has worked as a recreation therapist in general psychiatry for the past six years working with adults with severe chronic mental illness.

Cheryl Prediger graduated in 1988 from the University of Lethbridge with a Bachelor of Arts with a major in Recreation for Special Populations. Cheryl has been employed as a recreation therapist for five years at Alberta Hospital Edmonton and is currently overseeing the outpatient day program in the geriatric psychiatry program.

Janice Rachinski graduated from Centennial College in Toronto, Ontario, in Recreation Leadership. She received her specialization in recreation for special populations from Georgian College in Orilla, Ontario, in 1986. Janice is currently employed as a recreation therapist at Alberta Hospital Edmonton on the special assessment unit for patients with dual diagnosis. Janice has also been instrumental in initiating the development of community-based programs for individuals with mental illness through the partnership of a number of agencies.

Vicki Ryan obtained her Teaching Diploma in Adapted Physical Education from the Ulster College of Physical Education, Ulster University, Northern Ireland, in 1966. From 1966 to 1975 she taught physical education, health education and English to educationally challenged high school students in Northern Ireland and in Saskatchewan. Vicki joined Alberta Hospital Edmonton in 1975 as the Director of Recreation Therapy and she held this position until March 1994. Vicki's leadership in this position lead to the development of a recreation therapy department which is recognized as a leader in the field in Alberta and in Canada. Vicki's support and vision was instrumental in the completion of this extensive project.

Shelley Stasiuk graduated with a Bachelor's Degree in Recreation Studies from the University of Manitoba. She then worked in Winnipeg as a recreation therapist in long-term care and later at the Aberhart Hospital in Edmonton, with the spinal rehabilitation program. She began working as a recreation therapist in 1987 and later became a supervisor. Shelly is still working on the behavior modification program.

Sandra VanVlack graduated in 1993 with a Bachelor's Degree in Recreation and Leisure Studies from the University of Alberta. Sandy is currently completing her Master's degree in the same program. Since 1992 she has worked as a recreation therapy assistant in forensic psychiatry.

OTHER BOOKS FROM VENTURE PUBLISHING

The A•B•Cs of Behavior Change: Skills for Working with Behavior Problems in Nursing Homes
      by Margaret D. Cohn, Michael A. Smyer and Ann L. Horgas
Activity Experiences and Programming within Long-Term Care
      by Ted Tedrick and Elaine R. Green
The Activity Gourmet
      by Peggy Powers
Advanced Concepts for Geriatric Nursing Assistants
      by Carolyn A. McDonald
Adventure Education
      edited by John C. Miles and Simon Priest
Assessment: The Cornerstone of Activity Programs
      by Ruth Perschbacher
Behavior Modification in Therapeutic Recreation: An Introductory Learning Manual
      by John Dattilo and William D. Murphy
Benefits of Leisure
      edited by B. L. Driver, Perry J. Brown and George L. Peterson
Benefits of Recreation Research Update (1991-1994)
      by Judy M. Sefton and W. Kerry Mummery
Beyond Bingo: Innovative Programs for the New Senior
      by Sal Arrigo, Jr., Ann Lewis and Hank Mattimore
The Community Tourism Industry Imperative—The Necessity, The Opportunities, Its Potential
      by Uel Blank
Dimensions of Choice: A Qualitative Approach to Recreation, Parks, and Leisure Research
      by Karla A. Henderson
Evaluating Leisure Services: Making Enlightened Decisions
      by Karla A. Henderson with M. Deborah Bialeschki
Evaluation of Therapeutic Recreation Through Quality Assurance
      edited by Bob Riley
The Evolution of Leisure: Historical and Philosophical Perspectives
      by Thomas Goodale and Geoffrey Godbey
The Game Finder—A Leader's Guide to Great Activities
      by Annette C. Moore
Great Special Events and Activities
      by Annie Morton, Angie Prosser and Sue Spangler
Inclusive Leisure Services: Responding to the Rights of People with Disabilities
      by John Dattilo
Internships in Recreation and Leisure Services: A Practical Guide for Students
      by Edward E. Seagle, Jr., Ralph W. Smith and Lola M. Dalton
Interpretation of Cultural and Natural Resources
      by Douglas M. Knudson, Ted T. Cable and Larry Beck
Introduction to Leisure Services—7th Edition
      by H. Douglas Sessoms and Karla A. Henderson
Leadership and Administration of Outdoor Pursuits, Second Edition
      by Phyllis Ford and James Blanchard
Leisure And Family Fun (LAFF)
      by Mary Atteberry-Rogers
The Leisure Diagnostic Battery: Users Manual and Sample Forms
      by Peter A. Witt and Gary Ellis
Leisure Diagnostic Battery Computer Software
      by Gary Ellis and Peter A. Witt
Leisure Education: A Manual of Activities and Resources
      by Norma J. Stumbo and Steven R. Thompson

Other Books From Venture Publishing **117**

Leisure Education II: More Activities and Resources
        by Norma J. Stumbo
Leisure Education: Program Materials for Persons with Developmental Disabilities
        by Kenneth F. Joswiak
Leisure Education Program Planning: A Systematic Approach
        by John Dattilo and William D. Murphy
Leisure in Your Life: An Exploration, Fourth Edition
        by Geoffrey Godbey
A Leisure of One's Own: A Feminist Perspective on Women's Leisure
        by Karla Henderson, M. Deborah Bialeschki, Susan M. Shaw and Valeria J. Freysinger
Leisure Services in Canada: An Introduction
        by Mark S. Searle and Russell E. Brayley
Marketing for Parks, Recreation, and Leisure
        by Ellen L. O'Sullivan
Outdoor Recreation Management: Theory and Application, Third Edition
        by Alan Jubenville and Ben Twight
Planning Parks for People
        by John Hultsman, Richard L. Cottrell and Wendy Zales Hultsman
Private and Commercial Recreation
        edited by Arlin Epperson
The Process of Recreation Programming Theory and Technique, Third Edition
        by Patricia Farrell and Herberta M. Lundegren
Quality Management: Applications for Therapeutic Recreation
        edited by Bob Riley
Recreation and Leisure: Issues in an Era of Change, Third Edition
        edited by Thomas Goodale and Peter A. Witt
Recreation Economic Decisions: Comparing Benefits and Costs
        by Richard G. Walsh
Recreation Programming and Activities for Older Adults
        by Jerold E. Elliott and Judith A. Sorg-Elliott
Reference Manual for Writing Rehabilitation Therapy Treatment Plans
        by Penny Hogberg and Mary Johnson
Research in Therapeutic Recreation: Concepts and Methods
        edited by Marjorie J. Malkin and Christine Z. Howe
Risk Management in Therapeutic Recreation: A Component of Quality Assurance
        by Judith Voelkl
A Social History of Leisure Since 1600
        by Gary Cross
The Sociology of Leisure
        by John R. Kelly and Geoffrey Godbey
A Study Guide for National Certification in Therapeutic Recreation
        by Gerald O'Morrow and Ron Reynolds
Therapeutic Recreation: Cases and Exercises
        by Barbara C. Wilhite and M. Jean Keller
Therapeutic Recreation Protocol for Treatment of Substance Addictions
        by Rozanne W. Faulkner
A Training Manual for Americans With Disabilities Act Compliance in Parks and Recreation Settings
        by Carol Stensrud
Understanding Leisure and Recreation: Mapping the Past, Charting the Future
        edited by Edgar L. Jackson and Thomas L. Burton

Venture Publishing, Inc.
1999 Cato Avenue
State College, PA 16801